GLEVaman̄ 5 .00
'74

Computers in Medicine

Proceedings of the
Second International Symposium
held at
Blackburn College of Technology and Design
on 16th and 17th March, 1971

Edited by
J. Rose, M.SC., PH.D., F.R.I.C., F.I.L., M.B.I.M., M.INST.C.SC.

Director-General, World Organisation of
General Systems and Cybernetics

JOHN WRIGHT & SONS LTD.
1972

Distribution by Sole Agents:

United States of America: The Williams & Wilkins Company, Baltimore

Canada: The Macmillan Company of Canada Ltd., Toronto

ISBN 0 7236 0313 8

PRINTED IN GREAT BRITAIN BY HENRY LING LTD.,

A SUBSIDIARY OF JOHN WRIGHT & SONS LTD.,

AT THE DORSET PRESS, DORCHESTER, DORSET

PREFACE

THE Second International Symposium on 'Computers in Medicine' was held in March, 1971, at the Blackburn College of Technology and Design under the aegis of the World Organisation of General Systems and Cybernetics. A number of medical societies in this country and in America supported the Symposium presided over by The Lord Rosenheim, President of the Royal College of Physicians. This book is a record of the proceedings, lectures, and discussions, spread over four half-day sessions, the emphasis being on practical uses of computers in medicine. While the First International Symposium in 1968 dealt with areas of use (*where*), the second event was concerned with concrete applications (*how*).

Apart from the opening and closing addresses this book is divided into four parts representing the four sessions. The first part deals with a general survey of computer-based information systems in general practice and hospitals, while the three papers in the second part draw heavily on practical applications of computers to hospital case and clinical records. In the third part, the topics considered are applications in electrocardiography, patient monitoring, X-ray diagnosis, and clinical biochemistry. The fourth part deals with the use of computers in hospital administration and in marking medical examinations. Of particular value are the discussions at the end of lectures and the panel discussions at the end of the day's work. The emphasis is on critical appraisal of the realities of computer usage in medicine without the spurious and extravagant claims made by some in regard to the so-called 'omnipotence' of the machine.

I wish to record my sincere thanks to those who made the Symposium possible, particularly the deputy organiser, Dr. J. H. Mitchell, and the secretary, Miss R. R. Black. I am grateful to The Lord Rosenheim, who presided at the Symposium, to the four Chairmen of the sessions, and the lecturers for their kind assistance and helpful co-operation.

Blackburn, 1971   J. ROSE

The following Societies and Institutions have given invaluable support:

THE ROYAL SOCIETY OF MEDICINE

THE ROYAL COLLEGE OF SURGEONS OF ENGLAND

THE ROYAL COLLEGE OF GENERAL PRACTITIONERS

THE MEDICAL RESEARCH COUNCIL (U.K.)

THE ROYAL COLLEGE OF PHYSICIANS, EDINBURGH

THE BRITISH INSTITUTE OF RADIOLOGY

THE ROYAL COLLEGE OF SURGEONS, EDINBURGH

THE AMERICAN MEDICAL ASSOCIATION

THE ROYAL COLLEGE OF PHYSICIANS AND SURGEONS
    OF GLASGOW

CONTRIBUTORS

Professor M. R. Alderson, M.D., M.R.C.S., L.R.C.P.,
*Regional Cancer Epidemiology Unit, Christie Hospital, Manchester;
now at the University of Southampton.*

Professor J. Anderson, M.A., M.D., F.R.C.P.,
King's College Hospital Medical School, London.

Professor F. W. Donaldson,
*University of Tennessee Space Institute, Tullahoma, Tennessee,
U.S.A.*

A. Fleck, PH.D., B.SC., M.B., CH.B., A.R.I.C.,
Consultant Biochemist, Glasgow Royal Infirmary.

J. Emlyn Jones,
Regional Treasurer, Manchester Regional Hospital Board.

J. Hywel Jones, B.SC., M.D., M.R.C.S., L.R.C.P., M.R.C.PATH.,
Consultant Pathologist, Manchester Royal Infirmary.

F. Kennedy, F.R.C.S.,
University of Glasgow.

Professor T. D. V. Lawrie, B.SC., M.D., F.R.C.P. (Edin. and Glas.),
Walton Professor of Cardiology, Glasgow Royal Infirmary.

Professor B. Lennox, PH.D., M.D., F.R.F.P.S., F.R.C.P., F.R.C.PATH.,
Consultant Pathologist, Western Infirmary, Glasgow.

R. B. Marshall, B.SC.,
Systems Analyst, Western Regional Hospital Board, Glasgow.

J. H. Mitchell, M.D., M.R.C.P. (Edin. and Glas.), M.INST.C.SC.,
D.OBST.R.C.O.G.,
*Consultant Physician, Scotland; Joint Editor, International Journal
of Bio-Medical Computing.*

J. M. Rawles, B.SC., M.B., B.S.,
Woodend General Hospital, Aberdeen.

D. Reekie, B.SC., PH.D.,
Senior Physicist, Western Regional Hospital Board, Glasgow.

C. C. Spicer, M.R.C.S., L.R.C.P., F.R.S.M., F.S.S.,
Director, M.R.C. Computer Unit, London.

H. Summers, M.SC., M.B., CH.B.,
Barrister-at-Law, Department of Radiology, Manchester Royal Infirmary.

Agnes A. C. Wallace, B.SC.,
Western Infirmary, Glasgow.

B. D. Young, B.SC.,
Glasgow Royal Infirmary.

CONTENTS

OPENING ADDRESS BY THE PRESIDENT

The Lord M. L. Rosenheim, C.B.E., M.D.

President, the Royal College of Physicians

IT does not seem three years since the first Symposium on Computers in Medicine was held at this College. That Symposium was a resounding success and I have little doubt that this one will be too.

Dr. Rose has been indefatigable in organizing this meeting; the programme looks fascinating and now only I stand between you and those to whom you have come to listen. A comparison of the titles of contributions on the present programme and on that of 1968 shows what an advance in attitude has occurred. In 1968 techniques were largely discussed; this time we are to hear of complex practical applications of computers.

I am honoured and delighted, but somewhat surprised, to find myself President of the Symposium. I had better make it quite clear that, while I am most interested in the ever-growing number of ways in which the computer is infiltrating medical practice, and while I am full of admiration for those who understand the intricacies of computers and can actually talk to them, I make no pretence to understand the complex workings of present-day computing.

I do, of course, appreciate the role of the computer in Hospital Activity Analysis and the great value of the information so derived for hospital management. We are all becoming increasingly involved in management, whether we like or not, whether we are consultants or general practitioners, general physicians or pathologists. We must know about the needs of the district that we serve, the types of beds required, the waiting list and turnover time. It is quite evident that, in the future, the medical profession must either be prepared to administer or be administered. The computer is, of course, now firmly established in the laboratory, both the research laboratory and that devoted to routine services, and it is slowly edging its way into the recording of notes and even history taking.

My major scientific interest in computers lies in their use in renal disease and in the computer calculations that can be made from renal scans and flow measurements. In this, as in most specialties, the computer is daily adding to our knowledge.

An interesting and important development is about to occur in postgraduate and specialist education. Data will be regularly collected about the posts held and the ultimate aims of each young doctor in training so that it will be possible for the first time to get an overall picture of training in the National Health Service. The data can be compared with what is known about the probable needs for various specialists in the years to come and realistic advice can then be given to our young graduates. This is an exciting new use of computers.

There are now so many aspects of computing in medicine that I suspect that Dr. Rose is already planning a third Symposium. But now let us get on with the second and I have much pleasure in calling on Professor Whitehead to take the chair at the first session.

Computers in Medicine
SESSION 1

Chairman: Professor T. P. Whitehead

*Knowledge is of two kinds. We know a
subject ourselves, or we know where we
can find information upon it.*

SAMUEL JOHNSON

Use of computers in medicine

C. C. Spicer

INTRODUCTION

THE subject of medical computing is so wide and so technical that I obviously cannot cover it in a short talk. What I propose to do is to pick out some of the most important topics and in doing so I shall of course miss out some that others will think I should have included. I apologize in advance for this and hope that the more glaring examples will come up in subsequent discussion.

It will also be necessary for me to make a number of rather bald statements on controversial issues. Once again I hope that this will lead to discussion, preferably long and acrimonious discussion.

I propose to divide my talk roughly according to the three main classifications of the health services: preventive medicine and public health, hospital medicine, and general practice, and make some more general observations at the end.

PREVENTIVE MEDICINE AND PUBLIC HEALTH

This branch of medicine is generally considered somewhat less than glamorous but as far as medical computing is concerned I agree with Professor Alwyn Smith, who, in a recent meeting, said that it was one of the most successful areas of medical computing. Some of the reasons for this are obvious. Much of preventive

3

medicine is in fact concerned with problems of management and data processing and the mechanism for collecting and analysing statistics was already in existence. Furthermore the introduction of computers in this field involved no radical changes in existing patterns of thought. Generally speaking its main effect was to liberate the epidemiologist and the administrator from the need to confine their records to a size which could be fitted on to a single 80-column punch card and from the limitations of the conventional counter sorter. In addition to this the computer also allows them to make many more, and many more complicated, calculations than had ever been possible before: for example the computation of survival tables and statistical tests. Some idea of the type of public health problem which can be dealt with so satisfactorily by computer can be obtained from a consideration of notified congenital malformations. After the outbreak of malformations caused by thalidomide many countries, including this one, felt the need to introduce a continuous surveillance of the incidence of malformations with a view to detecting as early as possible a similar outbreak. This is a fairly considerable task on a national scale. It requires a continuous surveillance of the incidence of malformations of about 100 groups of malformations in about 150 local authority areas. It is also necessary to be able to compare the current incidence in each area with the general trend over the previous two or three months. When an upward trend is suspected it is necessary to carry out some kind of statistical or mathematical test on the data to see whether the trend is a real one or a statistical fluctuation. I think it is true to say that an adequate system for doing this would not be possible without the use of computers. I do not know the current state of the programme used for the purpose in this country but it was certainly sensitive enough to detect quite minor changes which were subsequently found to be caused by such administrative artefacts as the arrival of a new Health Visitor with a particular interest in congenital dislocation of the hip.

The setting up of a national medical record linkage system, whose value has been strongly urged by Dr. E. D. Acheson and others, would be quite unthinkable without the use of computers.

This type of surveillance is a routine task of any large-scale vital statistics office because a similar watch has to be kept on all kinds of disease trends and this can be rationalized and conducted much more rapidly with the aid of computers.

4

Another area in which the computer has, I think, proved its usefulness is in the work of the Medical Officer of Health. The best known example of this in England and Wales is the system introduced by Dr. Galloway in West Sussex. The problems of the Medical Officer of Health are very much those of management in general. For example the keeping of schedules of immunization and sending out reminders to general practitioners and patients of courses of inoculation and subsequent payments to the general practitioners are all problems of a kind familiar in industry. Similarly the administration of screening campaigns, such as those for cervical carcinoma, and the keeping of 'At Risk' registers present no new features to the computer programmer or to the Medical Officer of Health who is using a computer.

A field of preventive medicine in which the computer is essential, though the value of the operation as a whole is still somewhat controversial, is in very large-scale health screening of normal populations of the kind carried out by the Kaiser Permanente Organization in San Francisco, B.U.P.A. (U.K.), and in Sweden. Here the amount of data collected on each subject is extremely large, covering a wide range of physical signs and symptoms, past history, biochemical examinations, and X-rays. A high degree of mechanization has been introduced into its collection so that as far as possible data are directly recorded in the machine. The examination of these large amounts of data, covering perhaps two million people, is quite impossible without a computer and on the whole seems to have been computerized with singularly little trouble.

A growing field of application of computers in the field of preventive medicine which is perhaps less well-known than these is the use of mathematical models in the design and carrying out of prevention campaigns, particularly in underdeveloped countries. Many years ago Sir Ronald Ross himself suggested that the interaction between the malaria parasite, the mosquito, and the human being could be framed in mathematical terms and subsequently some attempts were made to solve the equations analytically. More recently the late Professor George Macdonald attempted to use a theoretical model in the field for the control of malaria, performing the very laborious calculations involved by hand. However, in the last few years before he died he was able to make use of computer facilities and by a very happy combination of field observations and computing was able to demonstrate the

5

value of this kind of approach in controlling the disease. Since this time similar models have been constructed of campaigns for the reduction of tuberculosis, leprosy, and enteric disease. It is too soon to judge the value of the more recent applications, but there is little doubt that the use of the computer will prove of value, though this may not be so in every case. The difficulty of this kind of large-scale model building is that if one has a reasonably flexible model and a sufficient number of adjustable constants it is possible to obtain good agreement between actual and predicted results even though the basic model is in fact totally erroneous. This is a very common situation not only in epidemiology but in almost any kind of large scale computer modelling.

HOSPITAL COMPUTING

I enter on this part of my talk with considerable trepidation, not only because it is a difficult and controversial field but also because it is one with which I have least personal experience.

Hospitals are so complex and so specialized in their operation that computer experience in other fields is often of little value. It is also very difficult, in a field so dominated by human values as medicine, to give quantitive estimates in cash terms of the benefits that might be or have been achieved by the introduction of a computer system.

The result of this is that a new, complicated system, of an experimental nature, difficult to justify in concrete terms, and probably requiring extensive re-organization of traditional procedures, has to be introduced into a professional environment notable for its conservative attitudes. There is clearly plenty of opportunity here for friction. Before going into the more controversial aspects there are a number of areas worth mentioning in which the computer has proved itself as a valuable aid.

Probably the best established of these is the use of computers in large clinical pathology laboratories. There seems to be rather general agreement that a computer is financially and otherwise justifiable in any laboratory handling more than about $\frac{1}{4}$ million specimens a year. A computer in these circumstances is not just a machine for doing arithmetic but a genuine aid to management.

Another application which is now firmly established, is the use of a computer for radiotherapy dosage planning. Here the computer is doing a calculation previously familiar and solved by approximate methods by hand.

Other direct applications of the computer occur in the management of acutely ill patients in intensive care wards and in controlling the complex machinery of modern anaesthesia. There seems to be some difference of opinion as to the true value of computerized intensive care. Possibly further work on the mathematical background will be fruitful.

Other applications will be discussed by other speakers and I do not wish to go into details but I would like to mention two examples that I find particularly interesting. One is the use of a computer in Aberdeen and Birmingham for recall of patients after thyroidectomy who show signs of thyroid deficiency. The other is the use of a computer by Professor Weir and his collaborators in Aberdeen to monitor the occurrence of adverse drug reactions. What I found very striking when I heard Dr. Weir's account was that the scheme required a radical overhaul of the whole system of recording prescribed drugs in the hospitals concerned, a not unusual sequel to computerization in any field. The thyroid follow-up programme has succeeded in reducing the work load by about 90 per cent by avoiding unnecessary recalls, and the method should be quite generally applicable to other diseases.

At the risk of offending those whose pet applications have not been mentioned I shall now go on to some of the more difficult and controversial topics of hospital computing. The central problem here is presented by the clinical record. There is, I think, a basic conflict between the highly structured formal type of record which is best suited for computer input and information retrieval, and the rather diffuse unstructured working document which is traditional. In addition, there is a natural reluctance to introduce or accept any system which adds another record to the clinician's clerical load.

I am not aware of any satisfactory solution or even of a universally accepted approach to the problems of deciding what items of this mass of material should be recorded and how. Existing or proposed schemes vary from a bare minimum record, such as a summary face-sheet, to the whole of the alphanumeric material relevant to the patient. The simplest systems are easy to introduce but are usually retrospective and contribute nothing to the care of the patient during his stay. The more ambitious schemes make heavy demands on the staff often without any sufficiently obvious return and are also very expensive in programming and computer resources. I do not think one can say more about the current situation than that it is still in a state of flux with no easy answers to the major problems.

The most interesting question of the current scene is undoubtedly the relative merit of systems of totally integrated hospital information making heavy use of on-line multi-access facilities and more modest schemes based on the gradual addition of separate hospital activities to the computer's repertoire. The controversy was brought to a head about a year ago by the publication of a report prepared by 'SCICON' for the Department of Health for Scotland and the Nuffield Provincial Hospitals Trust. This report concluded that the introduction of a highly integrated hospital system largely based on multi-access facilities would raise the price of computerizing a 500–600 bed hospital from about $£\frac{1}{4}-\frac{1}{2}$ million to about $£1$ million and it also maintained that the benefits of doing so would not be proportionate to the increased cost. Professor Anderson is reading a paper later and I hope that he and other speakers will comment on this question which seems to me a very important one at the present day. I am not in any sense an expert in this field, but I feel that 'SCICON' may well have over-estimated the price of introducing such systems on a national scale since a properly planned national policy could greatly reduce the cost of programming by standardization and probably also that of some hardware. I would also feel that the ultimate solution of the problem of the clinical record, if it is to be satisfactory to both the clinician and the computer specialist, must eventually rely to some extent on multi-access facilities. However the necessary programming and hardware is so expensive and so much development and research remains to be done that I do not see how this kind of system can be introduced on a large scale during the next five to ten years. The problem of cost is particularly urgent in this country since we can be quite certain that any National Health Service money which is spent on computers is money which will not be spent on something else in the health service and consequently it is most important to have clear advantages demonstrated for the more expensive system. I think it should be sufficiently obvious from such projects as space research and large weapons systems that there can be things which are quite simply too expensive for the British economy.

GENERAL PRACTICE

I have put in a section on general practice more from a sense of symmetry than because I feel that substantial progress is likely in the near future. General practice shares many of the difficulties of hospital computing while adding several more of its own, such as the geographical dispersion of the units, their general lack of administrative integration, and the difficulty of record keeping and retrieval in the conditions of a busy practice.

Many of the immediate problems of computerizing general practice could be solved—at a price. In the first of these meetings (February, 1968) Dr. Keith Bowden, who is working on experimental computer projects in general practice, supported by the Department of Health and Social Security (U.K.), gave a possible price of about 50–75 new pence per patient per year for a reasonably complete G.P. computer system based on multi-access facilities; I do not think any subsequent developments have altered this estimate significantly. As in the case of hospital computing the benefits of such a system must be judged against the uses to which the money might be put elsewhere in the general practice. It is to me rather a sobering thought that the record system is costing about as much per patient as the doctor himself.

A number of general practitioners have published accounts of actual or projected computer systems but I propose to mention here only that of Dr. C. Hodes, with which I am personally acquainted. This is a relatively simple system designed to recall patients for various screening procedures in a group practice with about 16,000 patients, using the local authority computer on a bureau basis. The expense of basic programming and computer time for such a system is not great, especially as the computer can be used at off-peak hours, but it involved a formidable amount of clerical work in setting up the basic records and appears also to require a half-time secretary on a day-to-day basis for handling the clerical work.

I would guess that general practitioners could get a very useful service by using computers on a bureau basis in this way without elaborate multi-access facilities. The extra clerical load in Dr. Hodes' system is certainly due in part to the special requirements of a screening service. The expense of programming could be greatly reduced if it was possible to develop a basic general practice package for some of the most commonly required

9

procedures such as making appointments. The most formidable problems would be encountered in transferring the existing records into a form acceptable to the computer.

An ideal solution would be for any large group practice to have its own computer, as Dinwoodie has suggested. But even if, as he proposed, such a computer sacrificed all Central Processing Unit elaboration for increase in memory size I would not visualize this as a financially practical solution for at least 10 years and even then it might be rendered obsolete by the advance of multi-access techniques. Possibly the whole process might be practical as part of a general reorganization of the Executive Council system.

GENERAL OBSERVATIONS

It is usual on these occasions to make some reference to future developments in computing. I only wish to make two points of this kind, one of which is that the cost of computing in terms of cost per machine instruction executed is likely to fall even further. The other is that the cost of programming these instructions has been rising since the introduction of computers and the rate of increase shows no sign of falling off.

The following figures which I obtained from a report of the Pan American Health Organization illustrate the situation very well:

Computing Cost per 100,000 Instructions (U.S. Dollars)		Cost of Preparing *One* Instruction (U.S. Dollars)	
1951	25·00	1951	4·50
1966	0·02	1966	6·00
1970	0·01	1970	7·00

To this may be added the facts that: (*a*) a trained programmer produces about five effective machine instructions per day, and (*b*) a complex on-line programming system may well contain up to 200,000 instructions, and require constant maintenance by skilled programmers after it is installed.

I think it is essential to make these points to an audience of which a substantial proportion are not computer specialists. At a recent meeting on medical multi-access computing no mention whatever was made of the considerable programming problems which arise in this kind of system.

Apart from these technical points there is the effect that computing is likely to have on the face of medicine itself.

About 10 years ago in a general article I made the not very profound remark that it was through the study of computer diagnosis that the most profound effects of computing would make themselves felt in medicine. This seems to me still quite true and the results are beginning to show in the number of fundamental articles on the nature of the diagnostic process by eminent physicians, prompted by computer applications. It is possible, as suggested by Professor Card and Professor Good, that the concept of a diagnosis as understood now may be by-passed by the mathematics in a direct progress from the symptoms and signs to recommendations for treatment. In any case the interaction between mathematicians and clinicians, such as that taking place in Glasgow, seems to me to be a distinct step forward in the progress of medicine, and likely to cause a considerable change in the philosophy and practice of medicine.

It is hardly necessary to say now that the computer, when it is told how to do it, can be quite an effective diagnostician. What I think is more interesting is the fact that it can do as well as it does with the very primitive mathematical tools that are available. For example, from the U.S.A., Italy, and Russia the computer has been reported as a useful aid in the diagnosis of certain types of congenital heart disease. All the computer programs used were based on a mathematical model which took no account of the clustering and correlation of symptoms. They would for example assume that temperature and pulse-rate were independent of one another.

Another mathematical technique which has been widely and effectively used is Discriminant Function analysis. This does at least take some account of correlations but its use in assessing relative probabilities and in selecting effective discriminating variables is certainly dependent upon, and may be critically dependent upon, the assumption that the variables have a known statistical distribution.

Difficulties of this kind will almost certainly be resolved by advances in mathematical technique. What is likely to affect the practice of medicine is that these and other new statistical techniques will have to be integrated into a sequential decision-making system quite different from anything so far used. I would also guess that there may be a move towards increasing use of physical signs more suited to mechanical than human sensory organs. In most medical applications the computer plays the role of a tool like the microscope. Information must be presented to it in a certain form for examination and if we are not careful we may find ourselves examining artefacts of preparation. Once the appropriate techniques have been developed the computer may well have as fundamental an effect on medicine as the microscope had in pathology.

DISCUSSION

Question (D. D. Rose): You spoke of Dr. Hodes' G.P. applications as being very cheap. Do you have any figures?

Answer: Actual programming cost was about £500; time was hired at cheap rates on the local authority computer at off-peak hours I think at about £20 per hour.

Question (D. D. Rose): What is the cost of using a computer per patient?

Answer: I was quoting Dr. Bowden's remarks at the first symposium in 1968 when he estimated the system in which he was working would cost about 50–75p (10/– to 15/–) per patient.

Comment (Dr K. T. Gruer): You mentioned the Guy's/Essex G.P. computer medical records project, and suggested a costing of 75p per patient per year. The system is a sophisticated on-line interactive system and not yet in a service mode, so that the quoted figure surely is a matter of guesswork.

In Livingstone, Scotland, a simple off-line batch processing system has been in a service mode for two years. The computer provides:—
a. A rapid index to the written records.
b. A surveillance and monitoring service (e.g., Immunization call-up, call-up for pre-school children for routine developmental examinations).
c. By-product of information for management and other purposes. Cost per patient is about 30p per year.

Comment (Professor B. Lennox): I hope this will be only one example of the way in which Scotland, where most work has started later than in England, is trying to benefit from experience of English mistakes!

Question (Dr. D. M. Goldberg): Has the Californian screening system run long enough to show that it saves money?

Answer: I do not think any detailed figures have been given. The possible benefits are discussed in the *Scientific American* for April, 1970, by S. R. Garfield, one of the Directors of the scheme.

Question (Dr. D. M. Goldberg): Is it possible to cost the benefits of the scheme?

Answer: Yes, but it is difficult. One may actually spend more money but produce better medical care for the patient, which is very difficult to cost in its own right.

Comment (Professor J. Anderson): It pays to keep examination alive even for a year. No real cost benefits.

On-line computing in the medical profession

F. W. Donaldson

INTRODUCTION

DURING the intervening three years since your last symposium, massive strides have been taken on computers in medicine compared to previous three-year periods. My files have become loaded with successes, and I am happy to say that a large percentage of the applications have been developed to the point where they have become on-line. But let me add that these advances in on-line time-sharing are still small compared to advances in the fields of finance and the scientific world.

Certainly we are all aware of the past reluctance on the part of medical personnel to jump onto the fast moving computer band wagon and this will probably be brought out again in this symposium. There is still much reluctance, but more and more members of the medical profession are learning that the computer is the only answer to the problem of stretching their services to provide the medical care that our enlightened society demands with the present and near future manpower limitations, and we in the computing field all realize that much more can be gotten from the computer by putting the medical profession on-line.

First I would like to indicate that on-line computing can hardly be separated from time-sharing and, at the expense of a possible time cut-off before the end of my main presentation, I would like to lay a bit of background on the subject of time-sharing since I am not sure of the background of my audience. Time-sharing is one of the reasons on-line computing is feasible from the standpoint of cost.

TIME-SHARING

DEFINITION

Time-sharing is a situation in which a number of computer users get together and share a single computer or possibly a group of computers. Thus time-sharing could be in the batch processing mode as in the early days of the service bureaux but today is generally considered to be the situation where each customer is on-line with a terminal of his own and thinks he is the only person using the machine. He calls up his own program and his data base from mass storage, does any modification necessary to his data base, such as updating it with new information, modifies his program parameters if necessary, and he is ready to start processing.

HISTORY OF TIME-SHARING

In the U.S.A. it is generally understood that time-sharing started with 'Project MAC' at the Massachusetts Institute of Technology where a number of schools in the Boston area shared the same computer. But I can tell you that before 'Project MAC' I was heading an effort developing time-sharing systems for the field army at Fort Huachuca, Arizona. We just didn't have a good publicity agent and also had security problems.

Commercial time-sharing came into its own in about 1966 in the U.S.A. when small companies got started on both coasts. Shortly after that a little company called General Electric got into the act!

ADVANTAGES OF TIME-SHARING

The chief advantage of time-sharing is that when a small company needs large computer capacity and can't afford a large computer of its own or even when the jobs are small but not enough in numbers to warrant the company having its own facility, the company can purchase time as needed and needs only relatively low cost terminals in its own facility. The real pay-off, though, is the situation in which a number of users of computers in widespread locations need to share a common data base. It may be impractical to duplicate the data base for all users and keep it updated in a number of different locations. A good example of this is where an atomic test facility is generating huge quantities of data and companies at great distance from the test site are using this data. It is better to have the data processed at the data location under remote control from the various company locations.

Time-Sharing in Medicine

Generally, time-sharing facilities solve problems from a variety of disciplines that are entirely disconnected. Time-sharing in the medical profession has a common goal or should have: improved, lower cost medical care. I would like to include some examples here. Medical applications are a natural time-sharing application because of the common data base; that is, a majority of applications in one locality share patient files and the users share a common computer or a common network of computers. However, there are medical applications which have a dedicated computer for a single application though the computer is operated on a time-sharing basis. An example is interpretation of E.C.G.s. Another is automation of blood chemistry (*Datamation*, 1969; *Proc. I.E.E.E.*, 1969). For example, if a doctor's office has a proper terminal attached to his E.C.G. equipment, he can input the signals directly into a dedicated facility which can interpret the E.C.G. and get a reading back almost instantly. One such computer facility (*Datamation*, 1969; *Proc. I.E.E.E.*, 1969) can interpret 1000 E.C.G.s per day with 1 per cent false negatives. A cardiologist can interpret a very definite negative in about three minutes, but if something is seriously wrong, it might take an hour. His false negatives might run as much as 10–15 per cent. If he went through all the gyrations that the computer program does, it would take him all day or longer for one. Hence time-sharing this facility by doctors over a wide area certainly makes sense and the cardiologist can be relieved to work on the cases found to be serious after the computer has uncovered them. In the case of blood chemistry, if a doctor can get 12 tests for the price of 3, why not? Automated laboratories are developing rapidly and are entirely on-line except for sample identity (*Datamation*, 1969; *Proc. I.E.E.E.*, 1969).

But now I am getting into everybody else's subject. Let me get into something different with hopefully as little overlap with the other topics on your programme as possible.

My paper is organized to start with what I consider the lowest element of medical care and proceed up the scale to the most sophisticated, pointing out on the way the turn to on-line time-sharing uses of the computer. All other professionals are taking advantage of on-line time-sharing. Why shouldn't the over-worked doctor take advantage of this means of relief?

MEDICAL QUESTIONNAIRE

We are now administering medical questionnaires under computer control with branching, and in cases where the patient cannot read for some reason (perhaps a language barrier or poor eyesight) the questions are asked in audio form in the patient's native language with push-button responses. The capture of patient profiles is of extreme value in the on-line administering of health care. Sophisticated procedures are available for file maintenance and rapid retrieval on a highly selective basis (Smith, 1970).

HEALTH SCREENING

We are all aware of the need for catching bodily disorders early enough to provide cures at the lowest level of the health service chain in order to conserve professional medical manpower. I am sure you are all familiar with the first effort in health screening in our country on a large scale, namely the Kaiser-Permanenti Multiphasic Health Screening in Oakland, California. In Dr. Maurice Collen's first efforts (Collen, 1967) data was collected automatically but largely on cards. Now with more than one-hundred such facilities in existence (*Computerworld*, 1969), many of which are mobile (Sherman, Bunow, and Yedidia, 1969; Yedidia, Bunow, and Muldavin, 1969), the trend is towards capturing test data on-line (Davies, 1969) with immediate computer analysis. Some tests reported appear after the patient's departure but this will not be the case for long.

Without going into detail on the on-line activities at the mobile and stationary health screening centres which will be treated elsewhere in your program, let us proceed to the next link of the health chain.

COMMUNITY HEALTH CENTRE

It is hard to treat this link of the chain without including the next link, the central community health facility, since they are tied together in the chain just as the health nurse is tied to the health screening stations via patient records. Let us picture the slum or low income area. Here the patient is entitled to the same health care as the affluent. Disease and poor health are no respecter of persons. In order to stretch medical care, health nurse's stations or community health centres are scattered at convenient intervals in these areas. The centres are on-line with a central medical facility. If the patient is ambulatory, he reports to the nearest centre. If he has a previous medical record, the nurse or clerk can retrieve appropriate files from this record by querying the central files. Answers to queries are returned immediately and printed on paper or displayed on C.R.T. If the patient has no medical record, one is started, possibly with the audio questionnaire on-line with the central facility, if the case is not an emergency. If so an abbreviated form is used. The usual information, such as temperature, blood-pressure, pulse-rate, etc., is gathered by the nurse and entered into the system. If the nurse can handle the case, such as in return visits or chronic cases, she does so. If she cannot, the first general practitioner available, or first specialist if the nurse so designates, at the central facility comes on-line in a video hookup to see the patient. The patient can see him. The doctor already has the patient record before him transmitted along with the request and shown him via the T.V. hookup. If he wants further tests that the nurse and assisting technicians or paramedical personnel can administer, he orders them and receives results on-line. These will include E.C.G. with computer interpretation and blood chemistry using *Auto-chemist** or equivalent with results transmitted directly to the physician hopefully on-line before the patient leaves. The doctor can take care of another patient in the interim while waiting for the completion of the tests. We must keep in mind that the nurse's station is handling a large volume of patients and elaborate equipment can be expected to be available with supporting technicians. *Auto-analysers** may be too costly for this level for some time.

If the doctor wishes to see the patient in person, he requests it and arrangements are made for transportation if the patient does not have his own. If the patient is sick at home, a mobile nurse's station moves to the patient's home and portable units are used to perform the same procedure as above.

THE CENTRAL FACILITY

The central facility is staffed with specialists and supporting paramedical personnel. The central processor for the service network is located here. The doctor makes maximum use of his time by treating his patients scattered among the nurse's stations via video hookup without leaving his oscilloscope. Patients can be

---

* Auto-chemists and Auto-analysers are trade names of the relevant analytical instruments.

scheduled to see the same doctor for each visit if desired, but this is held to a minimum for greater efficiency of the system. A general practitioner is first scheduled or nurse-collected symptoms could be fed into a specialist selection algorithm. If the case can be handled by the next doctor available, this will be done. He will signal his availability to the system when he is ready to see another patient. If the patient is sent to the central facility to see the doctor, of course he handles the case in the usual manner but he is equipped to do so at the location of his computer terminal or an adjacent examining room. Here more sophisticated examining equipment is located than at the nurse's station, but all readings from tests go directly into the central system for merging with the patient's file and at the same time displayed for the doctor to see. Of course, personal observations and summaries are dictated to clerical help either in person or via dictaphone for entry into patient files. If the patient is ordered to the hospital, admissions information is ordered from the patient's file by a clerk by instruction from the physician. He will dictate information for addition to the admissions information if required. The admissions record is then transmitted to the hospital ahead of the patient or is retrieved from the system at the hospital admissions desk upon his arrival.

All of the elements of the above concept are being tested at the present time. By the time you have your next symposium, a complete system should be in operation, if not more than one.

THE HOSPITAL INFORMATION SYSTEM

It is interesting to note that early efforts in medical applications of computers were attempts to implement total hospital systems. The job was bigger and more costly than we anticipated.

From the time the doctor prepares his hospital admissions information on a patient as retrieved (hopefully by the terminal of his receptionist or possibly his own terminal) from the patient's previous medical record supplemented by information on this particular illness, to the receipt of this information at the admissions desk, to the assignment of a bed, the scheduling of tests, the reporting of results, the ordering of medications, monitoring of administering medications, diet control, scheduling of operations, etc.—these are all on-line applications or should be. Information collection into patient files from these activities for business-type application is an on-line activity though the business applications themselves might be batch processed. Since this is a special topic on your programme, I will not go into further detail on this subject. However, I would like to indicate here that, in my opinion, the most valuable on-line application of the computer in the hospital to date is that of scheduling activities except possibly intensive care services. Our hardware manufacturers and software companies appear to be setting a strong pace in putting hospitals on-line. More efficient software modules are being put together for better total hospital systems.

Though the monitoring of radiation dosage (*Computerworld*, 1970) and the control of kidney machines (King, Baker, Ginn, and Frost, 1970) are not classed as intensive care, these are very important on-line treatment monitoring applications.

INTENSIVE CARE ACTIVITIES

These are taken up separately from the usual hospital systems because of their hybrid system nature. Here very sensitive instrumentation is attached to the patient, or in some instances the instrumentation is so sensitive that it need not be attached. The computer picks up the information, digitizes it where necessary, processes it, and sounds an alarm when vital signs exceed prescribed limits. The norms for comparison should be those established from the patient's previous medical history and such should exist and be retrievable. Otherwise a standard norm is used. The revising of norms should become a popular activity as well as the establishment of individual norms. In the intensive care ward the patient is on-line. Continuous recordings from instruments may be of extreme value to the doctor and are available for his viewing if needed for making new decisions.

THE PROFESSIONAL MEDICAL BUILDING

With the advent of the minicomputer and reasonably cheap terminals and mass storage devices, computers will be able to reach areas of the medical service chain that have never been reached before. Doctors are moving more and more towards group practice where specialists of all types are grouped together in one complex of offices and laboratories. Usually pharmacies are included. In my opinion this is a perfect set-up for implementation of my concept portrayed in my article in biomedical computing. The scheduling of patients to see the appropriate specialist is a valuable computer application. I will not go into detail here since you can read the article. At a very reasonable cost, the entire complex can be automated with all communications hard wired to the central facility which would occupy no more space than two examining rooms and cost less than one complete X-ray room. This system would have a linkage with the local hospital systems as indicated in my article. Except for putting the entire medical group on-line to a computer for greater efficiency and for added capabilities that would otherwise be impossible, there would be no change in the operation of the medical facility. Please note in my article that I do not propose that doctors and nurses use typewriters, though I would think that the doctor would be intrigued with the information retrieval capability that he could have at his C.R.T. terminal with the aid of a few chosen function keys. Light pens, or 'finger pointing', the Lockheed terminal, Sanders 708 display terminal, or Control Data Digiscribe* are ideal terminal types for doctor manipulation for diagnosis, medication, etc.

THE DOCTOR, LABORATORY, AND PHARMACY ON-LINE

Here again I must refer to my article in the *International Journal of Bio-Medical Computing* (Donaldson, 1970). The difference between this system and the environment of the professional medical building is that all three are separated, which makes hard wire communications without the use of common carriers impossible. Microwave communication is ideal in some settings. I would like to mention here that I know of at least one feasibility study going on at the present based on this concept. This is my own and it is nearing completion. There may be others. I will cover no more detail here unless you desire since the article is fairly detailed. Perhaps I should take this opportunity to mention here that my article was written four years before I was 'forced' to publish it. Were I to write it today, I certainly would not mention paper tape since tape cassettes had not become popular yet and I certainly would emphasize the rapidity of automation of laboratory instrumentation and the use of minicomputers.

MEDICAL RESEARCH

I would like to mention that the data base collected by the above on-line medical applications will be a valuable base for medical

---

* Trade name of Control Data Corporation.

research. Such data bases should be made available for use by medical researchers with patient identities withheld (*Computerworld*, 1970). With present fast information retrieval systems, the medical researcher could certainly do much of his file querying on-line. Files can be rapidly and selectively searched for statistical data.

PROGNOSIS AND DIAGNOSIS
I treat these together because of the similarity in at least one technique which I have chosen in hopes that I am not duplicating someone else's presentation. This technique has been used by the Veteran's Administration at New Haven, Connecticut (Feinstein, Rubinstein, and Ramshaw, 1969). In the same way that a weather man can use past weather profiles to predict weather, the doctor can use patient profiles compared to the nearest match of a similar case history from a huge data base as an aid to diagnosis and for prognosis. Again file search is so fast that the doctor can conduct his searches on-line. Here he will vary his search criteria to retrieve a manageable number of match case histories before having them printed out for making human judgement use of the files. This variation of parameters makes it desirable that he be on-line. For diagnosis, the doctor uses the case histories extracted as an aid in diagnosis. For prognosis, the doctor can determine the past best treatments, the chances of patient survival, etc., and these activities can be carried out on-line and in a reasonable length of time on the part of the doctor or medical researcher. No doubt diagnosis algorithms will be covered elsewhere in your programme and I will not cover the subject here. The use of computers as aids in diagnosis is still disappointingly low.

SOCIO-MEDICAL APPLICATIONS
In this type of application, the family is treated as a unit. Family medical records are kept together including other information such as education, positions held, government assistance, etc. Family planning might also be included in this application. A very workable system is in operation on the Papago Indian Reservation at Sells, Arizona. The reservation is very large, about the size of Connecticut, and has a sparse population of 5500. Of course, this system differs from the individual type only in that files may be queried by on-line terminals for family information when the case at hand warrants the information. This system may

very well become a prototype for other systems in our depressed areas where the family unit must be considered in the total health picture.

DOCTORS' CONTINUING EDUCATION

One bright spot in medical applications that looms over the horizon is that of keeping doctors updated by medical bulletins and by on-line query by the doctor. The busy doctor of today finds it extremely hard to keep up with his profession, as is the case with the rest of us. With page readers coming into popularity and the cheap transfer from journal to microfilm or microfische combined with the prediction of a 10,000-word spoken vocabulary, the doctor will soon be able to query the medical library and get immediate responses to his questions or have bulletins or articles either displayed on his T.V. screen for reading at his own speed or read to him by computer voice. When he queries the system for proper medications for a given disease, he is being automatically updated since someone will have the responsibility of keeping up to date these medications with appropriate dosages and possible side effects. The system described above can be used for continuing education for all medical personnel.

SUMMARY

In summary, the medical profession is finally going on the computer and a large part of the medical applications are on-line. It hasn't been easy. Many failures have been caused by attempts by hospitals to install systems using poorly qualified personnel in an attempt to save installation costs. The hardware manufacturers are now delivering very well designed systems, and some software companies specializing in medical information systems are likewise delivering a good product. Some insurance companies have been a driving force behind the progress in the United States. The large efforts have received government support. Though it has been a hard struggle for computer people to convince the medical profession of the value of the computer to them, I believe that within the next four or five years we will have most of the medical profession on-line. In closing, I would especially like to call your attention to a series of articles published in the May 1969 issue of *Datamation* and the Special Issue on Technology and Health Services, *Proceedings of the I.E.E.E.*, Nov. 1969. These series give very good summaries of the progress to those dates in medical applications of computers in the United States. We have come a long way since.

REFERENCES

COLLEN, M. F. (1967), 'The Multitest Laboratory in Health Care of the Future', *Hospitals*, **41,** 119.

Computerworld (1969), 'Milwaukee Medicine Program offers Free Tests to Over-40s', **3,** No. 20, 36.

— (1970), 'Cancer Treatment planned for Patients', **4,** No. 33, 6.

Datamation (1969), 'World of Medical EDP', Series of Articles, **15,** No. 5, 37–59.

DAVIES, M. (1969), 'Toward a Medical Data Bank for a Total Population', *Datamation*, Nov.

DONALDSON, F. W. (1970), 'The Doctor, Medical Laboratory, and Pharmacy On-Line', *Int. J. bio-med. Comput.*, **1,** No. 1, 1.

FEINSTEIN, A. R., RUBINSTEIN, J. F., and RAMSHAW, W. A. (1969), 'Estimating Prognosis with the Aid of a Conversational Computing Program', *Clin. Res.*, **17,** 477.

KING, P. H., BAKER, W. R., GINN, H. E., and FROST, A. B. (1970), 'Computer Optimization of Hemodialysis', *Int. J. bio-med. Comput.*, **1,** No. 4, 253.

Proc. I.E.E.E. (1969), Special Issue on Technology and Health Services, **57,** 1799–2042.

SHERMAN, S. R., BUNOW, M. A., and YEDIDIA, A. (1969), '"Computer Intervention" with People, Patients, and Physicians', Paper presented at the Medical Care Section of the American Public Health Association, 97th Annual Meeting, Philadelphia, Pa., Nov. 13, 1969.

SMITH, A. L. (1970), 'Algorithm-based Random Access Filing System Speeds Medical Aid for 1·5 Million Patients', *Data Process. Mag.*, 29–31.

YEDIDIA, A., BUNOW, M. A., and MULDAVIN, M. (1969), 'Mobile Multiphasic Health Screening in an Industrial Setting', *J. occup. Med.*, **11.**

DISCUSSION

Question (Dr. O. C. Parry-Jones): How much patient response has been investigated?

Answer: The systems have not been very long in operation, but the Boston General Hospital has had this facility for some time.

Question (Dr. R. J. Sims): These are imaginative schemes for maximizing the use of scarce expensive physician resources. One comment that may be allowed is 'God help the Doctors'. We know that the suicide rate for consultants over the age of 45 is well above that for members of the same social class in the general population of this country. Have you considered the possibility that the turnover of doctors will increase? The mental stress of making decisions about patients should not be underestimated. What studies are you undertaking to investigate the effect that the increased work load will have on the doctors?

Answer: No survey has been carried out of this problem. However, intensive computer usage is necessary, since this would assist poor patients (in the U.S.A.) to see a doctor. Also doctors may have less work to do because of medical automation.

Medical information systems

M. R. Alderson

INTRODUCTION

THIS paper discusses the use of Medical Information Systems for management purposes in the health service. A clear distinction must be made with systems handling medical information for direct use in patient care; such systems can be combined with a management system, as in a total integrated information system, (Lawton, 1970). I am restricting my attention to systems for the provision of accurate, comprehensive information for the effective control of work, and for the formulation of policy.

HISTORICAL BACKGROUND

The introduction of a system for collecting information about hospital patients was advocated as long ago as 1732 (*Lancet*, 1841). This country introduced a national scheme for processing vital statistics in 1838; however, it was not until Local Health Authorities took over management of hospitals in 1929 that interest reawakened, and large scale recording and analysis of hospital statistics began (Spear and Gould, 1936–7). The introduction of the National Health Service in 1948 provided the opportunity for the introduction of a national scheme for collecting hospital morbidity statistics. MacKay (1957) described the scheme and suggested that the data would be of value for management purposes. Benjamin (1965) drew attention to steps being taken to develop a basic information system for hospital departments. This system became known as 'Hospital Activity Analysis (H.A.A.)', the object of which was to feed back information to the hospital consultant about the operation of his department. Heasman (1968 and 1970) referred to a similar scheme in Scotland; the file of data was used to send information to each consultant about patients under his care discharged from hospital in the preceding year. At the same time, information was provided about the total work load for all consultants by particular specialty for each region

24

and for the country. Wall and Cross (1968) discussed the use of H.A.A. data in the Birmingham Region; they gave examples of how the data can be analysed to assist regional planning and to provide a basis for examining the work of hospitals. McNay (1969) reported experience in the use of H.A.A. in the Newcastle area; he emphasized that, partly due to the initial lack of computer time, the data was used primarily to investigate specific problems rather than produce routine output for transmission to all consultants in the region. *Ad hoc* analysis in response to specific planning or management problems had been used in the following three sub areas: (*a*) to assist long-term planning, (*b*) to assist in the evaluation of proposals for major changes in hospital provision, and (*c*) to assist in the evaluation of minor changes in provision or use of services within hospitals and within departments. Acheson in a series of papers has demonstrated how a hospital record linkage system can be used to monitor hospital management and identify areas for special study.

MEDICAL INFORMATION SYSTEMS

Bailey (1962) proposed adjusting the length of stay in response to changes in the length of a waiting list. He suggested, if the consultant in charge knew the exact state of affairs each day with regard to current waiting list, average length of stay, and turnover interval, that adequate control could be effected.

Weir and Crooks (1966) described a very restricted application of the development of medical information systems in Aberdeen. They referred to the standardization of hospital prescription sheets and the use of these forms to study the prescribing habits of different doctors, and the discrepancy between doses of medication ordered and doses given. They emphasized that the Aberdeen study was only a fraction of what was required, and they also pointed out that many parts and features of the medical records were in urgent need of similar analysis. Cross and Roberts (1970) discussed the fact that there is no accepted theoretical framework for medical management; they pointed out that a management information service must develop as a result of a dialogue between the data service chiefs and the managers themselves. This point was echoed by Nicholls (1970) who emphasized that management must define its information requirements and ensure that the relevant data is used in an effective manner. The same point was made by Downham and his colleagues (1969) when they spoke about information services for a management-by-objective programme in a psychiatric hospital. They pointed out that identifiable and measurable goals are required with definite points for starting and finishing the programme. Cross and Roberts reviewed the current systems available for providing management control; they were critical of H.A.A., stating that it is inappropriate for exploring medical management problems. They referred to the use of comparative studies, such as examination of the use of diagnostic resources by different clinicians. To date such comparisons have usually been carried out without thorough study of the objectives of the use of such resources. These authors drew attention to medical care review as carried out in some American hospitals; some attempts are made to assess effectiveness of hospital use, together with simultaneous measurement of quality of care. However, the objective of such American reviews, is to minimize the charge in an individual's episode of care; this is very different from the requirements in this country, where a more general examination of cost effectiveness and resources is needed. Cross and Roberts also mentioned the application of exception reporting, though the example that they give of this technique is the rather restricted one of signalling abnormal biochemistry results. Fairey (1970) stressed that managerial information should consist solely of exception reporting (i.e., specific reporting where the figure in any parameter deviates beyond the limits set by the administrator); he suggested that for management purposes real-time facilities will not be required. Dearden (1966), in a light-hearted article, concluded that real-time management information is a myth. Lawton (1970), in an article on a management orientated hospital information system, indicated that the prospect of data banks with detailed information captured routinely as a by-product of the day-to-day running of a real time system, was an exciting one for all staff who have managerial responsibilities. He did not spell out the specific use of this information for management purposes but was probably referring to functions which Fairey (1970) considered 'executive'. Keller (1969) suggested that today we have the means of making data available to all who need it in their role as individual decision makers, and that in a hospital this should decentralize the decision making function and free the organization from the constraints of a single decision maker. Elliott (1967) indicated that a Regional Board may be moving towards integrated management information with continuous and consistent

26

integration about patients, staff, resources, and money. Hopkin (1967), a consultant with the N.H.S., pointed out that unless those who write on this subject do so in less abstract terms than at present their message will remain meaningless and evoke no enthusiasm. This sentiment is echoed in the recent Civil Service Department Report, *Computers in Central Government Ten Years Ahead* (1971). This points out that although a copious amount has been, and is being, written about integrated management information systems these publications in the main scratch superficially across the surface of a complex subject. The report emphasizes the difficulties experienced both in industry and government in the setting up of integrated management information systems; they recommend that the best way of making progress will be by developing information systems on a small scale, at the same time providing for the greater build up of an integrated system.

CURRENT ATTITUDES TO MANAGEMENT IN THE N.H.S.

The recent report on the functions of the District General Hospital stresses that the best use will be made of specialized and expensive hospital facilities only if the community based services are seen to be capable of providing effective community care when hospital care is not really required. The report points out that it is easier to plan these services together, not separately. The first report of the joint working party on the organization of medical work in hospitals (Cogwheel Report, 1967) discussed how medical staff could become more involved in organizational problems. This report suggested that specialties should be grouped into divisions with the aim of reviewing hospital bed usage against the background of community needs, the organization of out-patient and in-patient services, and review of clinical practice. It was suggested that this would require a study of data on waiting lists, out-patient waiting times, and time spent in hospital by patients awaiting operation or investigation; the use of resources in terms of manpower and equipment should also be considered by divisions. It was pointed out that a system would be required for supplying relevant data in order for the divisions to achieve their functions. The report on senior nursing staff structure (Salmon Report, 1966) emphasized that the Chief Nursing Officer will have to develop effective channels of communication between nurses and other hospital officers and within the nursing service itself. It was felt that this was an important feature of the Chief Nursing Officer's job and necessary in order to obtain due consideration of proposals for better organization of the service.

The Department of Health and Social Security under the previous Government (1970) produced a second green paper on the future structure of the N.H.S. Unification of the health services was recommended with the formation of area health authorities and it was proposed that there would be a medical officer at area health board level who would be responsible for helping his colleagues monitor the need for and outcome from all clinical services. One of the main tasks of this 'community physician' would be to develop the quantity and quality of information about health needs and the working of area health services. It was hoped that the community physician would be able to take advantage of the new opportunities for collaboration through the system recommended in the Cogwheel Report.

THE WESSEX MEDICAL INFORMATION UNIT

It is against this background that a Medical Information Unit is being set up in the Wessex Region; this is a joint venture by the Regional Hospital Board and the University of Southampton, with half the financial costs being paid by the Department of Health and Social Security. The first task has been a review of information currently available in the health service, and the resources available for collection, processing, and analysis of this material. This has then been related to the areas of application of the data in order to clarify the uses to which the material may be put. The areas of application fall into three broad categories—administrative needs, medical studies, and teaching purposes.

The data will, we hope, help answer administrative queries at Board and Hospital Group level. These can be divided into problems dealing with three different time scales. First, some queries arise unexpectedly and require a relatively simple and quick analysis of current workload. Secondly, there is need for an annual stocktaking with examination of the unmet health demands of the population, the workload carried by the various medical and other staff, and the resources required to carry this workload. Thirdly, long-term planning requires precise information about current situation and anticipated changes in the future.

The routine data that is currently available is somewhat limited, and hard pressed to fulfil the above aims. Some of the day-to-day management problems can be readily answered when all they require is a tabulation of the current demand on or use of resources, plus perhaps simulation to demonstrate the effect of alternative forms of management intervention. However, many of the queries will relate to areas not covered at all, or in sufficient depth by the routine data collection system.

The difficulty with attempting a regular review of use of resources is that the simpler indices available from the data (such as turnover interval, bed occupancy, mean length of stay) can be very misleading. The doctor is the major determinant of the use of resources (once the patient has decided to contact the health service), and it is by no means sure that independent review of use of resources will in any way effect the behaviour of doctors. The divisional system introduced into hospitals is, however, a forum for the discussion of such data; we anticipate feeding to these divisions data which has been analysed as extensively as is possible, and is then presented in judicious quanta. We also hope that contact with doctors and administrators in the hospitals will foster the referral of requests for joint study of specific problems. Where the doctors are concerned about unmet demand, or deployment of resources, and instigate a special study, the findings are more likely to be translated into action, than to follow an independent examination of the material. Before conclusions are drawn about variation in the use of resources, the data must be examined from every possible angle, taking into account all the confounding variables. In many situations the only conclusion that may be drawn is that there is a need for collection of additional information, and more detailed study of the fresh material.

The routine data provides relatively limited information about the medical problems treated in hospital. The discharge data that is processed contain administrative and identification particulars, diagnosis, number and codes of operation performed, and fatality rates. Apart from crude numbers of first and subsequent attendances at out-patients by specialty, we have no routine data providing information about the reasons for attending out-patients, nor about the advice and treatment given. Some family doctors, particularly members of the Royal College of General Practitioners, collect information about the workload in general practice, with details of the diagnosis for which patients consult them, and the treatment provided. There is, however, no routine information available from general practice on this aspect. Analysis of the available data can therefore only provide a very limited picture of the current functioning of the health service. For planning one requires to know exactly what are the health needs of the population today, what health needs are translated into health demands, which of these demands are currently being met and how they are being met by the health service. This information must be related to the demographic characteristics of the population served. Knowing the anticipated changes in the basic population it is then possible to estimate future demands. One has, however, to take into account how the attitudes and requirements of the population may change in the future and how the family doctors and consultants in out-patients might alter their ways of handling patients such that dramatic changes in the requirements for resources occur. One thus wants to know for family doctors confronted with a particular condition not only what treatment he currently provides but what treatment or referral he might recommend if alternative facilities were available. Information is also required on innovations in treatment that are currently being tried so that one can foretell major changes in methods of delivering medical care. Finally, examination of trends in incidence and prevalence of disease must be studied in order to estimate the changes in health of the population that may occur independently of treatment.

This wide range of detail cannot be provided from a routine information system. The system has therefore to operate as a basic framework, providing limited information about current health care. The data should then be used as a sampling frame, so that *ad hoc* in depth studies can be mounted to explore many of the problems where change may occur in the future. One requires to build a conceptual model of the current functioning of the health service and build on to this the range of alternative changes in need, demand, and provision; from the model one can estimate, within broad margins of error, anticipated requirements in the way of staff and other facilities.

As already mentioned the medical data collected in the routine system are extremely limited and apart from providing a diagnostic index (of dubious accuracy) the requirements of clinicians interested in studying their own material requires considerable expansion of the system. It is essential that doctors, whether working in hospital or family practice, are provided with assistance should they have the enthusiasm to collect extended particulars about their own workload. Co-operating with clinicians in this way should improve the quality of the basic data; it may also help start a dialogue with clinicians which leads to management studies.

The final objective of the information system is to provide data for use in teaching. Initially, a diagnostic index will be provided; there will, however, be an increasing volume of material which throws light on the current functioning of the health service. This in itself may be useful to put any particular problem in perspective against the total health problems of a defined population. The data bank will serve as a framework for mounting epidemiological studies. Providing the system is capable of meeting the administrative and medical requirements, and can be made available for teaching purposes without breach of confidence, no additional facilities will have to be built into the basic system for teaching purposes.

Any routine data collection system is subject to problems of inaccuracy and inappropriateness of the basic data. We have commenced a limited study of the accuracy of our data. The results of this validation, together with further experience in the use of the material, will help us check the appropriateness of the items routinely collected.

This far I have said nothing about the use of computers, perhaps surprising at a conference on Computers in Medicine. The Information Unit will have to rely on computers for data processing, but the computing problems are small compared with problems of data collection, and definition of suitable areas of application of the material. Currently the computing requirements are modest—to handle a fairly large magnetic tape file off-line in batch processing mode. The main examination of the total file will be at regular but infrequent intervals; there is a need to examine sections of the file at irregular intervals and with a turn-round time of about a week. In course of time we shall no doubt identify gaps in our routine data collection system, and add further to the volume of input. Currently, each set of data relates to a single event during the course of the patient's life. We will have to face in due course the need to link successive events occurring to any particular individual. This will enable us to study long-term outcome of treatment, so necessary if we are to study use of resources in a meaningful way. Linkage will increase to a major extent the complexity of the computer system required.

REFERENCES

BAILEY, N. T. J. (1962), *Calculating the Scale of In-patient Accommodation Towards a Measure of Medical Care*. London: Oxford University Press.

BENJAMIN, B. (1965), 'Hospital Activity Analysis', *The Hospital*, May, 221.

CIVIL SERVICE DEPARTMENT, MANAGEMENT STUDIES 2 (1971), *Computers in Central Government Ten Years Ahead*. London: H.M.S.O.

COGWHEEL REPORT (1967), *A First Report of the Joint Working Party on the Organization of Medical Work in Hospitals*. London: H.M.S.O.

CROSS, K. W., and ROBERTS, J. L. (1970), 'Management Controls in Medical Care', *The Hospital*, **66,** 45, 81, 121.

DEARDEN, J. (1966), 'Myth of Real Time Management Information', *Harvard Business Review*, May–June, 123.

DEPARTMENT OF HEALTH AND SOCIAL SECURITY (1970), *The Future Structure of the National Health Service*. London: H.M.S.O.

— — — — CENTRAL HEALTH SERVICES COUNCIL (1967), *The Functioning of the District General Hospital*. London: H.M.S.O.

DOWNHAM, D. J. (1969), 'Information Services for a Management by Objectives Programme in a Psychiatric Hospital', *Nursing Times*, May, 569.

ELLIOT, J. (1967), 'The Hospital Clinician's Role—As a Hospital Administrator sees it', *Lancet*, **2,** 1248.

FAIREY, M. J. (1970), 'Information Systems in Hospital Administration', in *Medical Computing—Progress and Problems* (ed. ABRAMS, M. E.), pp. 384–389. London: Chatto & Windus.

HEASMAN, M. A. (1968), 'Scottish Hospital In-patient Statistics', *Hlth Bull., Dep. Hlth Scotl.*, **26,** 4.

— — (1970), 'Scottish Consultant Review of In-patient Statistics', *Scott. med. J.*, **15,** 386.

HOPKIN, D. A. B. (1967), 'Doctor as Manager', *Lancet*, **2,** 1417.

KELLER, T. F. (1969), 'The Hospital Information System', *Hosp. Electronic Data Processing J.*, 170.

LAWTON, M. D. (1970), 'Systems Design for a Management Orientated Hospital Information System', in *Medical Computing—Progress and Problems* (ed. ABRAMS, M. E.), pp. 358–359. London: Chatto & Windus.

LEADING ARTICLE (1841), *Lancet*, 649.

MACKAY, D. (1957), *Hospital Morbidity Statistics, G.R.O. Studies on Medical and Population Subjects No. 4*. London: H.M.S.O.

MCNAY, R. A. (1969), 'Hospital Activity Analysis', *The Hospital*, 308.

SALMON REPORT (1966). MINISTRY OF HEALTH AND SCOTTISH HOME AND HEALTH DEPARTMENT (1966), *Report of the Committee on Senior Nursing Staff Structure*. London: H.M.S.O.

NICHOLLS, R. M. (1970), *Management of Medical Resources in Resources in Management*. (King Edward VII Hospital Fund, London.)

SPEAR, B. E., and GOULD, C. A. (1936–7), 'Mechanical Tabulation of Hospital Records', *Proc. R. Soc. Med.*, **30,** 633.

WALL, M., and CROSS, K. W. (1968), 'Recording and Analysis of In-patient Data on a Regional Basis', *The Hospital*, **64,** 354.

WEIR, R. D., and CROOKS, J. (1966), 'The Development of Medical Information Systems', *The Medical Record*, **7,** 311.

DISCUSSION

Following Professor Alderson's lecture the Chairman referred to the problem of accuracy of data obtained in laboratory analyses, particularly since the results obtained varied with the technique used.

Answer (Professor M. R. Alderson): I agree that the accuracy of data must be carefully studied. As regards dissemination of information, we do not favour producing lots of computer output and sending this round the region. Having done an analysis we hope to telephone the doctors concerned and visit them to discuss the problems.

Question (P. T. S. Brown): Was automatic analysis better than the manual one?

Answer (Professor T. P. Whitehead): The autolyser has produced better results. Because of automation larger laboratories do better.

Question (D. C. Manley): The trouble is that the larger laboratories do not believe they are wrong. How do you deal with this?

Answer (Professor T. P. Whitehead): We are working on it.

Question (Dr. R. J. Sims): In the collection of data for activity analysis the central problem is to stimulate the interest of consultants so that one can get reliable data on diagnoses. In East Anglia we have tried to find, without success, an application for H.A.A. that consultants can use regularly on a day-to-day or week-to-week basis. We have even asked other Boards if they were aware of such an application but without success. I wonder if Professor Alderson has any ideas in this direction?

Answer: Computers can only edit data; they cannot validate them, and we are mounting a separate validation study. There is a difficulty in processing management data; it is little use processing routine data and showing what is already known. But if doctors come with problems, the data can be analysed and this is likely to result in action, and change in the situation.

Question (Professor J. Anderson): What are the results of the validation?

Answer: We have only just got going on this. Work I did elsewhere showed the administrative data were accurate, but the diagnostic data were less so.

Information flow in hospitals

J. H. Mitchell

INTRODUCTION

BEFORE introducing computers into clinical practice in hospitals we should examine in detail the present state of information handling there. Otherwise we shall aggravate an already disorganized situation.

A great many of the irritations of everyday life arise through defects in the communication of information. This is both surprising and alarming when we remember the growing complexity of factual data in our technological society, and the necessity for increasing exactitude when systems are computerized.

Herein lies the reason for the change in recent years in the general public's attitude towards computers. At first it was one of wondrous admiration; now it is one of cynical hostility. The use of these machines has resulted in a sharp deterioration in customer satisfaction in retail shops, in the nationalized fuel industries, and in insurance and income tax transactions. This is because of poor systems analysis, but the computer is blamed by its users when inefficiency is challenged by the customer. It is, after all, far easier to blame a machine than a person when things go wrong, and the general *depersonalization* of a system is the most pernicious side-effect of computerization.

> *I know a bank wherein computers whirr,*
> *Where customers no longer merit 'sir'.*
> *Where electronic tellers twist your name*
> *Into a sort of tortuous numbers game;*
> *Which, with your status, pride, your very soul*
> *Is fed into some grim magnetic hole,*
> *Till you've become, with no chance of escape,*
> *A brief statistic on a piece of tape.*

(RAYMONDE, 1970a)

THE HOSPITAL NETWORK

Viewed as an information network any large hospital today is in a chaotic state, and we must beware of compounding this chaos by computerization. Two significant news items reached the columns of one of our highly respectable national papers last year. The first was a humorous, rather than harmful, example of *ambiguity*: an extract of a Hospital Management Committee report which read as follows:—

> 'The admission of both sexes to a single ward has resulted in far better use being made of the beds and has not produced practical difficulties.'
>
> (PETERBOROUGH, 1970a)

The second item, by contrast, was an account of an extremely serious case of *misplaced identity*. The headline (*Daily Telegraph*, 1970) read, 'Doctor accused of shotgun medicine', and the text related how, at a Coroner's inquest, it transpired that an 86-year-old woman had been admitted to hospital and mistakenly matched with the case records of a younger woman of the same name who was on the waiting list for admission and who was on maintenance therapy with tolbutamide. The patient in question was then treated with tolbutamide for 6 days before the mistake was discovered, and she subsequently died in coma.

It is essential at this point to stress that the problem is not restricted to aspects of case record format and storage; it concerns all aspects of information handling, and is therefore one of cybernetics. The greatest obstacle today to the efficient practice of medicine is the difficulty of rapid and accurate communication of known facts about individual patients between one doctor (and/or nurse, and/or technician) and another (e.g., *see* Levitt, 1969).

A somewhat analogous situation in industrial and business management has attracted the attention of cyberneticians in recent years (Cook, 1970). In medicine, however, the real cost of this kind of inefficiency is measured in human morbidity and mortality rather than in financial units.

The flow of clinical information in hospital can be represented in a geographical fashion (*Fig.* 1), or, in more detail, in terms of the case records themselves (*Fig.* 2). This network can be immediately and greatly improved by attention to details of case record format and storage, medical secretarial organization, electro-mechanical recording devices, telephones and document transportation, but I have discussed these in detail elsewhere (Mitchell, 1969) and do not propose to do so again now.

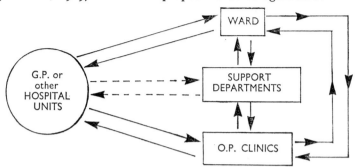

Fig. 1.—Flow of clinical information (geographical framework). Support Departments include laboratories, X-ray, E.C.G., E.E.G., physiotherapy, etc.

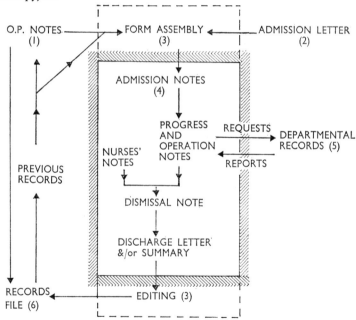

Fig. 2.—Flow of clinical information (case records). Locations: (1) O.P. Clinic; (2) G.P. or other Hospital Unit; (3) Ward or Records Department; (4) Ward; (5) Laboratories, etc.; (6) Records Department.

The question we must at present consider is whether computerization at any point is indicated; not, be it noted, whether it is feasible.

COMPUTERIZED DATA BANKS

One of the basic aims in work study is to merge as many tasks as possible into one operation, like the way one factorizes an algebraic equation. It follows logically, therefore, that all the various indexes which are at present kept separately in a hospital (e.g., master, morbidity, diagnostic, and operation indexes) would be better computerized to form the basis of an admission/discharge and registration bureau, which, in turn, would attend to mechanical documentation. Suitable software already exists, because airline companies have used computerized reservation systems for a number of years; in fact these companies have been forced to computerize to remain economically viable (Davis, 1970).

The inevitable temptation to extend the scope and size of such a computerized data bank for no very good reason (the syndrome of 'digital madness') must be firmly resisted. For example, the increasingly complex hospital activity analysis of in-patients which is operated by the Scottish Home and Health Department is, to my mind, already quite unreasonably demanding of the precious time of nurses and medical secretaries, who have to complete complex questionnaires for data input.

Problems of *taxonomy* and *semantics* arise frequently when data abstract forms are used to supply data banks. Technical terms may be incomprehensible or simply misleading.

'"Good morning, madam," said the young man on the doorstep of a Sussex housewife. "Are you converted?"
"Well, actually," she replied, "I'm a practising Anglican." "I'm from the gas board," he said.'

(PETERBOROUGH, 1970b)

Confusion may be due to the wording of the form itself, and the form filler is sometimes expected to draw conclusions which are by no means obvious. For instance, 'occupation' may mean occupation of husband or father although such is not stated.

'An office boy newly engaged by a London professional body was instructed to stamp its official seal on letters received for departmental heads. He did so on an elegant parchment from Buckingham Palace congratulating the institution on its achievements. Reproved for it, he replied: "How was I to know where it was from? It was just signed 'Elizabeth' with no surname"'.

(PETERBOROUGH, 1969)

CASE RECORDS

Any attempt to computerize case records themselves, for diagnostic or other reasons, immediately poses problems of *standardization*. Diagnostic scoring from data lists remains useful in particular situations, as can be seen from the popularity in Japan. of the Sano Haematoma Index (*World Medicine*, 1970), but in general clinicians quite rightly refuse to be organized into interrogating and examining patients in a standard fashion as if they were simply faulty engineering equipment.

To take a specific example, even though I personally set about obtaining certain routine information (laboratory facilities permitting) as a first step when investigating a patient's hypertension (*Fig.* 3), I know very well that few other clinicians would choose to proceed in *exactly* the same way. Clinical evidence is collected, as is evidence in criminology, in order to argue a case, not to assemble a finite jigsaw puzzle. Medical practice is full of 'ifs' and 'buts' which cannot be resolved by standard search trees. To quote Browne and Freeling (1967):—

> *The only assumption that the doctor is entitled to make about the purpose of a consultation is that the patient is making a communication to him. The purpose of communication is not merely the conveying of information (informative) but to initiate certain actions by the doctor (promotive) and to produce feelings in the doctor (evocative). Moreover, it is not merely the words the patient uses which are the substance of the information; every nuance of expression and action is relevant. Nothing in the content of the consultation is accidental, although it may be unintentional.*

Serial B.P. readings.

Hb, M.C.H.C., total and differential W.B.C., blood film, E.S.R.

Serum urea, electrolytes (including calcium), cholesterol, proteins.

E.C.G.

Chest X-ray, I.V.P.

Routine urinalysis, M.S.U. microscopy and culture, water concentration and dilution tests.

Urinary catecholamines, 17-keto- and 17-ketogenic steroids.

Fig. 3—Preliminary investigations in a case of hypertension.

Even the task of recording clinical information on a visual display unit on each and every patient-occasion is so much more difficult and time-consuming than hand-writing an entry in a paper case record that it seems to me to be a non-starter; quite apart from the fact that on-line access to a computer would be necessary for 24 hours of every day of the year.

DISCHARGE LETTERS

It has often been suggested that at least hospital discharge letters could be easily standardized. I would disagree here also, having had experience of the standard letter form used in Aberdeen Teaching Hospitals. In some instances the relevant data can indeed be set out in a straightforward list manner, but in most it is virtually impossible thus to convey sufficient information, and each letter must become a 'one-off' document. Otherwise the burden of drawing significant and correct conclusions is transferred from the sender to the recipient, and, moreover, the account may be so tidied up that it has what Richard Asher (1958) called 'the dullness of a sieved diet'.

Before I am contradicted on this point let me quote one such non-standard letter:—

13th August 19—

To patient's G.P.; copy to Consultant Obstetrician.
Dear Dr. ——,
> Patient's name and address: 21 yrs, housewife.
> Transferred from Obstetric Unit 7th August;
> for discharge home tomorrow.
> Diagnosis: 1. Normal puerperium.
> 2. Drug dermatitis.

Your patient was delivered of a male child on 6th August. The placenta had to be manually removed but blood-loss was not marked. She had had diarrhoea at home two weeks previously, for which, I understand, you had prescribed phthalylsulphathiazole; on the day before delivery she had a short recurrence of diarrhoea, hence her transfer to this Unit.

She had no further diarrhoea and rectal swab cultures are negative.

On admission here she had an intense non-itchy purpuric eruption on neck and shoulders, which I think was a drug rash. It subsided spontaneously. The following are known to be possibly responsible:—'Pethilorfan', morphine, atropine, ergometrine, pentobarbitone, crystalline penicillin and sulphadimidine.

The latter two drugs were given in the Obstetric Unit for one day before transfer, but she had no chemotherapy thereafter.

Breast milk has been suppressed, at her request, with the usual doses of stilboestrol. The child is quite healthy, but has not yet had B.C.G.; his mother is keen that he should have this, so perhaps you would make the arrangements.

Her Hb 10·1 was g% on 7th August, and ferrous sulphate has been started in a dose of 3 gr. t.i.d.

Yours sincerely,

That text is such an intimate admixture of narrative and comment that its essentials could not be adequately and succinctly set out in list form.

CONCLUSION

Although I am an enthusiastic supporter of computerization where it is appropriate, I think it is very important to keep a balanced view by playing the role of devil's advocate from time to time. Moreover I have considerable sympathy with the views of the poet already quoted, who also wrote (Raymonde, 1970b):—

> *Here I stand, a little child,*
> *Computed, classified and filed,*
> *Taped and indexed though I be,*
> *Here I raise my hands to thee,*
> *For a thunderbolt to fall*
> *On Data Maniacs one and all.*

REFERENCES

ASHER, R. (1958), 'Why are Medical Journals so Dull?', *Br. med. J.*, **2,** 502.

BROWNE, K., and FREELING, P. (1967), *The Doctor-Patient Relationship.* Edinburgh: Livingstone.

COOK, W. A. (1970), 'Cybernetics: the Key to Industrial Communication Efficiency', *J. Inst. computer Sci.*, **1,** 66.

Daily Telegraph (July 11, 1970).

DAVIS, H. G. (1970), 'Computers—a Means of Survival', *J. Inst. computer Sci.*, **1,** 46.

LEVITT, H. N. (1969), 'Hospital Letters', *Br. med. J.*, **3,** 594.

MITCHELL, J. H. (1969), *A New Look at Hospital Case Records.* London: Lewis.

PETERBOROUGH (1969), 'London Day by Day', *Daily Telegraph*, March 12.

— (1970a), *Ibid.*, Aug. 7.

— (1970b), *Ibid.*, Dec. 1.

RAYMONDE (1970a), 'Your Number's Up', *Rancid Rhymes, Sunday Telegraph*, May 31.

— (1970b), 'It's a Blessing', *Ibid.*, Oct. 18.

World Medicine (1970), 'Add up Your Diagnosis', **6,** 1, 46.

SESSION 2

Chairman: Professor J. G. Scadding

*One of the greatest pains to human nature
is the pain of a new idea.*

WALTER BAGEHOT

'Switch'—hospital case history on computer

F. Kennedy

THIS paper describes our experience in introducing a computer system to handle the case records of patients attending the Peptic Ulcer Clinic and the Department of Surgery at the Western Infirmary, Glasgow. The system was conceived in response to a specific need, namely to organize clinical information collected during the routine management of patients in a manner that would simplify subsequent research evaluation.

PEPTIC ULCER CLINIC

This clinic is held once weekly and is run by the Department of Surgery as a routine service to the hospital. About 470 new patients per annum are referred by general practitioners or by other hospital specialists. The majority are referred to be considered for surgical treatment of peptic ulcer while some have post-gastric surgery problems. About 200 patients are subsequently admitted for operation and thereafter assessed at regular intervals at the same clinic. Clinical information relating to these surgically treated patients is of particular interest for research. Some clearly defined research projects already exist, such as a random trial to compare vagotomy and gastro-enterostomy with vagotomy and pyloroplasty (Kennedy, Gillespie, and Kay, 1968). Other investigations will involve prolonged follow-up and correlation of the results of surgery with intra-operative and pre-operative factors.

41

A computer system was sought with the following requirements:—

1. It should handle all the clinical information available on peptic ulcer patients whether collected for routine management or for research. This should also include data of apparently limited potential research value in case it should be of future significance.

2. The system should interfere as little as possible with the existing clinical management and administrative structure, and should be acceptable to its users, the clinicians.

3. Flexibility should exist so that the nature and amount of clinical data recorded were not rigidly fixed.

4. The system should be reliable and accurate.

5. The cost, although not precisely delineated, should be practical for a teaching hospital.

When these requirements were studied, it became evident that the problem had much in common with the more general problem of computerizing hospital case records. This wider development was considered in devising a system not only to serve the specific needs of peptic ulcer research, but also to serve as a pilot study in handling hospital case records by computer.

'SWITCH'

The expense of an on-line computer system was not economically justifiable nor was such a system necessary, and so a batch processing system, 'Switch', was devised. This has been described in more detail elsewhere (Kennedy, Cleary, Roy, and Kay, 1968) and has been in full operation since September, 1967. Information from the out-patient clinics, the operating theatres, the wards, the routine hospital service departments, and the research laboratories is collected on 11 different documents.

CLINICAL DATA

The data collected during routine examination and management is not normally in the highly organized form most suitable to computer storage and manipulation. Some organization of this data was necessary. One could organize data in a 'fixed format' such as a check-list or series of 'yes–no' questions. Variable length lists of items may be required. The completely free format of conversational English is necessary in some areas. The documents were designed in a mixture of fixed and variable format, of precisely defined data fields, check lists, lists of varying complexity and sections of free comment.

Within this complex framework, three types of information are allowed: (1) Numeric or coded; (2) Dictionary items; (3) Free comment.

There is no difficulty with numeric or coded data. Heights, weights, and the results of many laboratory investigations are already in numeric form. The severity of symptoms can readily be coded from o to 3. To indicate the accuracy of some of the data, item modifiers were introduced. These can indicate that a piece of information is 100, 75, 50, or only 25 per cent reliable in accuracy. These item modifiers are stored by the computer and can be used later in statistical weighting of analysis.

Some items require code lists too large to be conveniently used while collecting clinical material. It would be impractical to use the 'International Classification of Diseases' to code diagnosis while interviewing a patient. The computer maintains a dictionary of clinical terms and uses this dictionary to replace in store the alphabetic terms used by clinicians with the corresponding code numbers. This dictionary handles terms from five categories, symptoms, treatment, diagnosis, operations, and physical signs, and will soon be extended to include investigations. The dictionary is flexible so that coding can be altered when required and so that new terms can be handled automatically. The dictionary originally contained 2500 terms and now three years later contains over 5000 terms. No attempt has been made to constrain clinicians to use particular terms in a deliberate attempt to assess the range of synonyms in common use.

Free comment is allowed on documents and forms an essential part of any routine case history. This deals with information which does not fit the standard framework or permits the expression of opinions perhaps of short-term value only. Such comments can be stored and reproduced by the computer, but are not readily analysed.

DATA PREPARATION

From the documents, data must be converted into a form readable by the computer. This is done by punching eight-hole paper tape on programmatic flexowriters (*Friden Limited*) in the hospital computer department. These instruments can be considered as sophisticated electric typewriters which, on keying information, produce both typed and paper tape copies. To minimize errors at this stage documents are punched separately in duplicate and other automatic features prevent errors of sequence in punching. Our experience suggests that any errors that do arise are due to misinterpretation by operators of hand-written medical terms. A project under way at present will assess the accuracy of the system by studying 40,000 extracted items.

COMPUTER PROGRAMS

Paper tape containing all the clinical information collected on documents is processed at least once weekly by a suite of programs written for the KDF9 computer in the Department of Computing of Glasgow University. The programs have been written in Usercode to utilize the time-sharing system and require six magnetic tape decks, 20,000 words of core store, and 1 million words on disc. The suite of programs was written and tested by programmers employed by the Department of Surgery on research grants, and the in-put programs were completed in about 3 man-years. There are five programs in the suite.

1. *Case Sheet.* This produces an on-line print-out on hospital stationery of certain documents particularly of those arising in the out-patient clinics. These are inserted routinely in the hospital case records.

2. *Data Vet.* Checks for errors in range or format and separates the dictionary items from the rest of the data.

3. *Dictionary.* This up-dates the dictionary file on magnetic tape with new terms and replacements and then replaces the dictionary items of data with the appropriate code numbers.

4. *Cross-reference.* Updates a dictionary cross-reference file maintained on magnetic tape with a reference to the occurrence of all dictionary items within the patient data file. This is necessary to allow flexibility in altering the dictionary structure.

5. *Input Up-date.* Simply merges again the output from 'Data vet' and 'Cross-reference' to produce a patient up-date file.

6. *Patient Master Up-date.* Using the patient up-date file the patient data file receives new patients and extra data for existing patients. This file holds patient's data sequentially and at present data from 9300 documents are contained on one magnetic tape reel.

The programming effort mentioned above does not include the provision of extract programs to take out and analyse information from the patient data file. The original intention was to use a general extract program which, when provided with detailed

44

parameters, could extract any required information in a particular format. Because of the varied forms of the in-put documents, it was found that specification of extract parameters was too complicated to be carried out by clinicians untrained in mathematics. A change of policy now provides that programs are specially written for each specific extract requirement. Several such programs have already been used to extract information of administrative value within the system and a program to extract 250 items of information of clinical importance from each of 350 patients is currently being tested.

FLEXIBILITY

In designing the system, consideration was given to the need for flexibility so that documents could be altered or new documents produced if required with a minimum of expenditure of time and effort. This flexibility was achieved by designing 26 general sections of different shapes handling different types of clinical data. Documents were then constructed using these sections as building blocks, and, with further flexibility within these sections, new documents can readily be constructed. The programs are written in a modular form around these general sections so that extra documents can be introduced with no additional programming effort.

This has allowed a more general expansion of the system into other clinical areas and the Glasgow Blood Pressure Clinic, meeting in four Glasgow hospitals, now feeds information into the 'Switch' system with a completely different set of documents.

COST

Such computer systems demand detailed cost-benefit assessment. It is too early to assess the benefit of 'Switch', since its value in peptic ulcer research will not accrue until at least five years of patient follow-up have elapsed, and its true role as a pilot study in hospital case record computerization is not yet elucidated. However, it is possible to be more precise about the cost. Research grants from various sources, in particular from the Nuffield Provincial Hospitals Trust and the Scottish Hospital Endowment Research Trust, have allowed the employment of programming staff, the purchase of technical advice from English Electric Computers Limited, the purchase of data processing equipment, and the salaries of operating staff. Making no allowance for the considerable time and effort provided by permanent members of the Department of Surgery, but allowing an estimate for the cost of computer time provided free by the University Department of Computing, 'Switch' has cost about £25,000 to develop over four years.

Although expansion and development of the system continues, an estimate can be made of current running costs. To include three flexowriter operators with depreciation on machines, one full-time programmer, a part-time medical editor to provide essential liaison between clinicians and computer staff, and estimating the cost of equivalent time on the University computer, £9000 per annum would be required to run 'Switch' only for peptic ulcer patients. This is less than £20 per new patient per year.

CONCLUSION

At present 'Switch' has been running routinely for peptic ulcer patients for over three years and we have on store case records relating to 1500 patients. We are satisfied that in-put of current detailed clinical information is practical and extension into other clinical fields is being proved in the Blood Pressure Clinic. Our current efforts are directed towards proving the accuracy of stored data and evaluating the difficulties in extracting a large volume of information of clinical relevance.

REFERENCES

KENNEDY, F., CLEARY, J. J., ROY, A. D., and KAY, A. W. (1968), '"Switch"—A System producing a Full Hospital Case History on Computer', *Lancet*, **2**, 1230.

KENNEDY, F., GILLESPIE, I. E., and KAY A. W. (1968), 'Comparison of Pyloroplasty and Gastrojejunostomy', *Gut*, **9**, 734.

DISCUSSION

Question (*M. P. Mansfield*): What system do you use for identifying patients ?

Answer: We give each patient a unique identifying number within the system which is not related to other identifying numbers such as hospital records number.

Question (*Professor F. W. Donaldson*): Is your extract program designed to prevent research workers from obtaining the identity of patients ?

Answer: No. There is no limit on access by research workers since at present all research is carried on by clinicians within our own Department of Surgery.

Question (*Dr. H. Summers*): Are there any benefits accruing from this work, or is it just a research project?

Answer: The main benefits are in the field of research, but there are extra benefits in managing our patients in that more information is routinely collected and the print-out gives more easily accessible presentation of an out-patient visit. There is one worrying disadvantage of using these stylised documents and that is that we are concerned that undergraduate and postgraduate students might assume that this is the only satisfactory method of taking a peptic ulcer history.

Question (*Dr. A. Fernandez*): How does one manage data that cannot be put in a numerical form? Do you input to your system only digital data via flexowriters or do you also input non-numerical information as radiographs, etc.?

Answer: Our system only caters for Alpha numeric information.

Question (*Dr. O. C. Parry-Jones*): How many lines of research have you pursued?

Answer: At the moment most of our resources are being used to carry out clinical research, particularly on patients being followed up after surgical treatment. However, some other lines are being followed such as assessing the errors within the system and looking at observer variation in collecting the data.

Computerized system for clinical records

J. Anderson

IN proposing a computerized system to deal with clinical records a case still has to be made that a change in the method of dealing with clinical records is necessary. Few doctors and nurses, because they have grown up with the existing pen and paper system, realize its difficulties and drawbacks for it appears to be infinitely flexible, although the medical defence associations would agree that at times it is less than adequate in providing a basis on which investigations can proceed as to what happened at any particular time. This emphasizes the difficulties in completing documentation where there is lack of standardization and where there are problems of record retrieval. At any one time at least some 10 or more per cent of medical records are missing when required and a few per cent seem to be permanently lost in any record system. Thus entries are often not made in records, because they are not available. Clinical records also include data of the communications established about a patient with investigative and therapeutic departments. Most laboratories would agree that about 10 per cent of the analyses carried out never reach the bedside although they are performed on specimens provided by the patient's doctor or the patient himself. Thus there are deficiencies in the communications system for ensuring that information which is created about a patient reaches the doctor at the bedside who ordered the investigation and who is responsible for interpreting it for patient's clinical care.

Existing hand-written records too are very difficult to analyse, and there are many errors in the documents. To proceed with analysis, it is necessary to transcribe records onto other documents and to encode these. The free format of the written text makes any such analysis extremely difficult except by rather laborious techniques, using a computer. As a communications document the existing record is inefficient and better systems need to be designed to ensure that what is ordered at the bedside is in fact carried out, and the results received by the doctors, and used to guide patient care. More efficient means of communication in the large modern hospitals and between general practitioners and hospital laboratories has to be established to ensure that there is neither waste of resources nor duplication of work because of deficiencies in the execution of requests and in the communication system. Increasingly as the demand for medical management increases, the need to make better use of existing resources remains. Medical records must be analysed for these purposes. Further information from medical records is essential to control general administration in both group practices and hospital. There is a need that requirements be met by using the basic clinical data in different ways so that information can be derived for management and administrative purposes, and so simplify the task of predicting and optimizing the utilization of resources.

With the growth and development of medicine, there is no doubt that in future there will be an increasing data load for analysis. Already the number of investigations done on patients has increased by several hundred per cent in the last decade and shows no sign of slackening. With each advance in the physical sciences go advances in both investigative and therapeutic medicine. As both investigation and treatment become more complex the number of variables to be dealt with by the clinician increases. This rapidly increasing number of facts to be considered becomes beyond the abilities of the ordinary man's memory or a pen and paper system. In future we will have to use tools that assist man in his analysis of large amounts of information. It will also be useful to see that routine tasks are carried through to completion automatically.

It is envisaged that new models of disease based on control systems will gradually develop in many areas of medicine over the next decade and clinical records are required to match this kind of model. These cannot be on pen and paper systems but require a tool such as the computer which will enable data to be analysed soon after it is available so that it can be used as a monitor of the patient's progress. It is likely that a new integration of medicine can come through computerized records when a great deal more knowledge will be available, about existing disease. The individual memory of any one doctor will no longer become so important, but the memory of the tool he is using will advance his capabilities.

49

The areas in which control systems seem likely to develop seem to be those of the control of the on-going energy system of the body and its associated disorders, the control of the system of what is 'self' and 'non-self', both in relation to infections and cancer, and also in the emotional and social field of what is self, the associated group and others. Undoubtedly in future the contribution made by pre-programming of life pathways due to genetic and family influences will become much more fully understood. A great deal of preventive work will take place on the basis of genetic tendencies which can be modified by altering the environment of the patient. Thus one can see the need for different kinds of data from a multiplicity of areas to be made available in future. For this, new tools will be required both to ensure analysis and on-going control in medical disorders by computer techniques, both actual and latent. Already this type of control has been shown to be valid and useful in the field of prophylactic immunization. It will extend without doubt into the fields of prophylactic diet and other type of treatment within the next two decades. Computerized records are becoming a necessity because the existing system of medicine is outgrowing its recording tools.

In designing a computerized system of clinical records, it is important that the objectives of this system be carefully defined and available to all who are taking part. These are extremely difficult to design. It is difficult to get an agreement about the implications of new tools which as yet are not fully understood by the ordinary physician and doctor, nor is their potential appreciated because the existing systems are familiar and their defects are not necessarily recognized as being unacceptable in future. The objectives for the King's College Hospital will be published elsewhere (Anderson, Crocker, Hedley, and Jones, 1971) and it is important that these be appreciated by all taking part in designing and implementing a computerized system.

The objectives are developed in a hierarchial system so that all the detailed objectives are included within those attained at an overall level. The overall objective is to create and maintain a complete patient medical record for life, including the medical records made by the general practitioner as well as by hospital physicians, nurses, paramedical, medical, and administrative personnel. This would represent an on-going record of a fixed format but at variable length accessible in part or on occasions in the whole. It should be emphasized that access to the whole data base should be rare and that interposed between the total medical record data would be a series of summaries designed to provide different types of information at different levels of detail. Thus, for information that is required urgently and frequently by the user, there can be early and rapid retrieval. Also, to meet the need for the occasional search, there can be much more information provided with the penalty that with the increasing size of the record, there is less accessibility in time. Thus a computer record system so designed could respond to different kinds of user demand flexibly.

The total medical record so created would be available for research into disease and disease patterns as well as being fundamentally designed for the optimal pattern of patient management and treatment within the given medical knowledge at a particular time. It would also be used for medicolegal purposes, for medical management and administration, and also for management of the health service as a whole. This implies that not only will doctors in the hospitals and the community nurses contribute to the medical record but a great number of different types of doctor throughout the whole of the patient's life. Paramedical personnel will also be responsible for much information in it, especially for that dealing with investigative departments, and in the therapeutic area.

Quite a lot of information is of a temporary nature and would require deletion, but some information will be permanent in the medical record. It is therefore important to ensure not only systems for promoting accuracy and direct identification of patients with information but also systems for erasing temporary information at various stages and so to decrease the necessary information that has to be stored. It is anticipated that a great deal of information would be transferred to various summaries and hence reduce the access to the total data bank. It is envisaged that the total medical record would not be available until the late seventies or early eighties, but its forerunner would be an on-going hospital clinical record covering the medical events for particular patients. It is anticipated that this basic clinical record of episodes of illness would be available for some patients in 1971 and would, with the development of adequate archive systems, be extended to the hospital in 1972 and beyond.

The development of analytical procedures of medical records once the data base and methods of input are adequate, will enlarge the potential of the doctor for investigating and treating patients and improve the ordering and communication processes. It is anticipated that such changes would bring changes in medical practice, freeing the doctor from many of the routine medical chores and give him more time to both work with his new tool and to improve patient care. It would also give facility of error checking both in the clinical and communications field to a much higher degree than is available at present. A reduction in error rates at present is absolutely essential if the recorded data is to be used for control and prediction in the clinical area. These overall objectives are the basis on which detailed objectives are made at four levels and developed into objectives which can be studied by systems analysts and implemented in the development of a computer system.

At the detailed level, methods of recording require to be investigated and decisions made about what is acceptable both at present and in the future in both recording procedures and in presentation of data to all who are concerned with the medical record. There have been many arguments about how data is to be entered into the computer and who should read various kinds of data, and these issues will now be raised. It is important to realize that data should be able to be entered into a computer system in a variety of ways, either by real time communication by means of codes or of free text into a computer or by entry remote from the user at a terminal, by punched input from data previously recorded by ordinary pen methods, by optical character recognition devices and by tape from a teletypewriter. Thus it should be possible for any computerized system to take a whole variety of input derived in a great variety of ways which will suit the user and can be used to make the clinical record. It has to be realized, however, that records which have to be encoded and punched up, take a considerable amount of time to reach the main computer record and therefore will not be incorporated rapidly into the total patient medical record. Thus they cannot be interrogated rapidly and may put a delay on use and analysis in this respect.

In general there has been a lack of flexibility in the approach as to who records data for entry to the computer system, and the type of record required. In Sweden they have tended to use operators who operate visual display units using a code-operated recording system. They are used because they are thought to be more accurate than medical people, and because the system uses operation codes, known in the main only to operators who translate documents. Unfortunately each transfer of information from one person to another not only allows errors to be transmitted, but also tends to create errors itself in the system. Thus it is preferable that the many individuals who originate data should enter it straight into the system. In the King's College project, this aspect was considered to be of paramount importance. Errors tend to be less if they can be checked visually when entered and translation errors therefore do not arise. However, the type of computer system to operate both real and batch time is more complex than that required just to use a batch mode of entry. It therefore costs more to create.

While it is important for input to be carefully planned and flexible it is necessary for output to be variable in its presentation. It should be possible for users to interrogate the system on demand, while having their access restricted by means of entry codes. Printed output should be available for those who wish to consult the whole of a patient's record and this can be temporary and either renewed everyday or several times a week as required, and then destroyed when the patient leaves the system. At present in the King's College Hospital project, we are filing the computer notes with the ordinary patient notes so that there will be no disruption in the hospital record system until it has been totally superseded. Thus the means of interrogating what has been recorded can also be flexible either in the short-term with interrogation of a visual display unit or teletypewriter or by printed records of varying sorts. A variety of people will read these records which are confidential.

In the communications procedures system with investigative laboratories, radiology departments and also with service departments supplying treatment such as physiotherapy, a large number of paramedical personnel will have to receive orders from the computer system originated either by doctors or nurses and carry out procedures either on specimens of patient's secretions or patients in response to these orders. The computer system will be responsible for booking facilities and ensuring that the process is carried through. The records so created will be checked by the computer system before being entered into the patient's medical file and will then become available for interrogation. Thus the computer will not only establish and book communications between investigative and therapeutic departments and patient's medical advisers, but also do some error checking and guide the procedure through. At this kind of activity, computer systems are far more reliable than ordinary hand procedures. It is not realized that in many laboratories about 10 per cent of the work done never reaches the patient's bedside due to wrong identification of patients or specimens. To increase the throughput and the accuracy of investigative and therapeutic departments, it is essential to develop new systems involving computers. It will also increase the reliability of data and the loss of information to patients by reducing errors both of omission and commission.

In designing the medical record there will obviously have to be format rules which define the content and the boundaries of any area to be recorded. In recording information about a reality it is necessary to see the information through some kind of framework or from a viewpoint so that the content of what is being observed can be recorded and only that aspect of the total reality which is being observed. In disease there is a great deal that is not relevant medically and it is necessary only to record the necessary relevant medical facts. Thus, formulating rules and discipline about what is to be entered into the system require to be determined and laid down so that all who use the system can understand them; only then will recording be satisfactory. A computer system has no real intelligence in the sense that it can transfer experience from one area to another and thus the persons who record the data have to do this kind of checking and observation of rules if the data is to be analysed adequately. Error checking procedures too in computers depend on the correct information being entered into the correct area, otherwise the analysis will not proceed satisfactorily without a great deal more programming effort.

Definitions have to be created of what is the content of the present history of the patient's illness and define also what is expected in the past history, social and occupational histories. The format and extent of the physical examination have to be defined so that a variety of types of physical examination can be conducted in various circumstances in relation to various disorders. If some compulsory minimum data is required then this must also be specified so that the computer system can ensure that this is obtained. Again in describing areas of provisional diagnosis and patient management, specifications of the various types of entry are required. Thus, if nurses are to use the system, nursing orders and nursing comments must be entered into specific areas and then the system can check that orders are carried out and that comments are noted.

Because the data in the system is more accurate and free from errors and follows a known format, analysis becomes much more easy than hitherto. As the data is structured it can be decided what types of user require what types of data and so this can fairly easily be collected. In general, the analysis of medical data tends to proceed on a temporal basis, following the natural progress of a disorder and the restoration of health. However, it is also easy to use the same data in a real-time computer system in quite another way for management purposes. As every item has a time of entry it is possible to take a cross-section of the whole activity of a ward or to study particular areas of a hospital at a moment in time and so derive useful medical management and administrative data from such an analysis.

It is not appreciated too that analysis of data by the computer system during the patient's illness may be extremely useful when a large amount of data have to be scanned and several logical procedures undertaken. Experiments are beginning at King's College Hospital now to investigate the application of a critical path analysis in scheduling the stay of a patient who has one of the common disorders. This enables critical investigations to be done at known times in the patient's stay. Checks can be made that these are carried through and appropriate actions taken as a result of the information derived from the investigation. It is possible to optimize investigative and therapeutic activity during a patient's stay and to keep this to the optimum that is required. We are tending to view the stay of the patient in hospital as a control system that can be brought under surveyance, and by means of adequate pre-programming and analysis of data, kept on an optimum path.

Such activities as these do bring forward problems of medical management where decisions about investigation and treatment can be decided in general before the patient's admission and certain critical pathways determined. Thus a great deal of ordinary routine care can be pre-charted and only exceptions allowed to influence the course. It is possible for the consultant to keep things on-line very easily when the computer system can help in part with the checking. We have also found it useful not only to have printout on the wards but printout for the consultant elsewhere so that before he comes to see the patients he can check the information out and decide the problems. It is thus possible to make more efficient use of medical time and clinical care by means of a planned dissemination of information, at predetermined times.

To date we have found the total patient record system quite difficult to develop, largely because of difficulties in attitudes of junior doctors and because it does take somewhat longer to enter data into the computer system than using a pen and paper method. Some of this increase in time spent entering data is not because of problems in typing or in encoding data, but because the system does tend to lead the doctor to a greater depth of analysis than is usually expected when recording an ordinary history by pen and paper. We have had problems of presentation of data in our system and even now it is far from perfect. It is slowly improving all the time as we experiment with newer and better ways of presenting existing data. The problem of presenting summaries of the total data to various users is receiving attention so that the whole record need not be consulted every time a problem arises. It is important to develop better and larger summarizing procedures so that a great variety of information is available for different people without necessarily accessing the total record of any one patient.

It would be wrong to give the impression that all of this computerized system of clinical record has the approval of most of the consultants in the hospital. This is not so. They feel that the existing system is adequate and so far do not appreciate the errors to which the existing system gives rise. In fact, some of them have declared that it is perfect. However, about 20 per cent of our records are missing when needed at any one time and some 3 to 4 per cent are permanently lost in the system. We have difficulties with communication procedures between investigative areas and the wards, and some 10 to 20 per cent of information never reaches the patient's bedside. It is not appreciated that errors of interpretation in the various investigative departments can be quite high, of the order of 20 or 30 per cent, and this has been well documented in the radiological literature.

Clinical errors do occur and clinical records have their errors. So far this aspect has been little investigated. Only one study in relation to circumcision has revealed that clinical interpretation of data may vary as much as 30 per cent although this study in itself had its own errors and therefore was not absolute (Lilienfield and Graham, 1958). We are now undertaking such an investigation on the observations made by doctors in the Medical Unit to try and determine the kind of errors that are likely to be incorporated into the recording systems, and allow for this in designing algorithms to interpret data.

In designing the computerized system of clinical records a firm decision was made early in the course of the study, that the implementation would proceed on a test bed area which was to be the Medical Unit, before the whole project expanded to other areas in the hospital. This technique has proved invaluable for many of the difficulties have been borne by doctors, nurses, and others in a limited area of the hospital, without being inflicted on all. It has, however, meant that many individuals in the hospital have not taken a great deal of interest in the project and are, at times, quite unaware of what progress has taken place. Education is slow; although it is offered it is not necessarily accepted.

We have found students, nurses, and paramedical staff, on the whole, much more interested in the new system of recording than the senior medical staff. There are problems of educating personnel in hospital and outside. We run repeated courses for our own staff to ensure that they can use the peripheral equipment and appreciate the advantages the system has to offer. There are educational problems too in relation to systems analysts and programmers, for the medical type of system to be analysed is strange to them for many come from computer projects in a business environment. It may take some 3–6 months for them to be thoroughly familiar with the hospital environment to understand its vocabulary and different ways of working. There are many problems relating to developing a computerized system for clinical records in a hospital. So far, however, these are not insuperable and we will be without pen and paper records on the test bed area within a month.

REFERENCES

ANDERSON, J., CROCKER, N., HEDLEY, R., and JONES, B. (1971), in the press.
LILIENFIELD, A. M., and GRAHAM, M. S. (1958), 'The Validity of Determining Circumcision Status by Questionnaire as Related to Epidemiological Studies of Cancer of the Cervix', *J. natn. Cancer Inst.*, **21**, 713.

DISCUSSION

Question (J. E. Fisher): Would you do it again the same way ?

    Answer: Roughly yes, but I'd insist on a signed contract when buying hardware to get what is really needed. I would also pay better salaries to the systems and programming personnel, since they have displayed great loyalty and devotion. I would also not regret time spent with students; it pays dividends in the long term.

Question (Professor M. R. Alderson): Since waiting list methods are not successful, I cannot see why you do not use peg-board systems.

    Answer: Because the bed state is updated at midnight. Hand-driven systems are not up-to-date because there is no amending system over the 24-hour period. One hopes that in a real-time information system updating would take place frequently as patients were discharged and errors would not occur. The 24-hour update would then be a check on the whole procedure.

Question (Dr. J. H. Mitchell): How do you record clinical data ? Do you use check lists ?

    Answer: The display system at King's College Hospital works by the user interrogating a series of displays organized as a branching questionnaire. There are several thousand displays in the system. As a result of interrogating these displays, messages are formed and displayed for verification when the end of a tree is reached. Once verified and given a numerical value between 1 and 9 to indicate their clinical importance they are stored in the patient's medical record. The display system is based on three main types of display; 'P' displays offering a single choice to descend trees, 'Q' displays give more than once choice allowing for descriptors for statements, the 'R' displays allow numbers to be inserted into a fixed format for reports, etc. This system meets the needs of about 60 per cent of medical recording. The demand-response system allows orders to be entered into the system and is a means of correlating orders issued by doctors, and responses by investigative and therapeutic departments. This deals without 20 per cent more of medical recording and is the main activity in the communications systems. We accept all types of input including free text, so that the system is flexible to changing demand. We are now working on the use of patient questionnaires to speed the entry of history data into the system and so lessen the information entry load on junior doctors, consultants, and registrars in out-patients.

Question (Dr. E. T. Gruer): Are you convinced—I am certainly not—that clinicians and nursing staff will be prepared to input information via a visual display unit and call up information via a succession of frames ? It seems that such techniques of history taking must be taught to medical students. What is your view ?

    Answer: It is very easy to learn to use the visual display unit. The incentive to use it depends on the returns the user gets from the system. These are greater initially for the nurses than the doctors. Junior doctors of necessity record far more information than they use. They do have problems of input in the experimental system in the past. It is expected that these will be largely overcome by the end of April this year. Some of the problems were anticipated before they occurred but it is not always possible to convince committees that problems will exist. Patient questionnaires will help to solve some of the problems in history taking. By having an on-going patient record much recapitulation will be unnecessary as summaries will be available. All students at King's are now being taught about computers in medicine.

Question (J. R. Brooke): Could you give me some idea of the cost of hardware you think would be required for a complete installation similar to that being developed at King's College Hospital and the time that would be required to develop such an installation?

Answer: This is a difficult problem, as hardware and software costs alter with time and demands. I would have thought that the hardware cost of a system with 60 visual display units and a failed-safe system for a hospital of 600–700 beds would cost about £500,000–£600,000. For our group of 2000 beds some £800,000 would be the hardware cost for five hospitals. Software costs are of the same order over a 5 to 7-year period. Thus, for something just over a million pounds, it is possible to get a complete hospital information and communication system which will create certain savings. In Sweden administration costs at all levels absorbs about 10–15 per cent of a hospital budget. Our annual budget is nearly £8,000,000 at King's. Thus in one year alone the administrative chores done by the computer mean that we can afford at least £500,000 to meet this demand. This would pay for a computer system in the long term. However, medicine itself will change to meet new techniques so I see little saving in the long term, in reality. The increased costs of such a development taking place in the existing system would be too great to be carried. A hospital information system could be implemented within 5–7 years.

The application of numerical taxonomy to the separation of colonic inflammatory disease

J. Hywel Jones

IN this paper I am going to talk about how patients may be arranged into disease groups. This process is analogous to the broader biological problem of classifying animals or plants and new techniques in biology can usefully be applied to medical classification. One such technique is numerical taxonomy (Sokal and Sneath, 1963), a quantitative method of classification which is useful when the distinctions between groups are difficult because each group lacks a defining characteristic common to all its members. The non-specific types of colitis are an example of a situation of this type in medicine.

DEFINITION OF DISEASE

There are two kinds of biological classification and these have been labelled by Sneath (1962) as 'monothetic' and 'polythetic'. Monothetic groups are defined on the basis of a single character or a set of single characters and to qualify as a member of the group an organism must have this character. A polythetic system of classification, on the other hand, places together organisms that have the greatest number of shared features and no single feature is necessary for being a member of any special group.

In the classification of disease both monothetic and polythetic systems are useful. A few years ago Scadding (1967) wrote an interesting article in which he explained how a disease may have a defining characteristic and this is essentially what I am referring to now as monothetic classification. For example, in phenylketonuria the defining characteristic is deficiency of the enzyme phenylalanine hydroxylase, while in tuberculosis it is the presence of the tubercle bacillus. The defining feature is not necessarily the aetiological agent: it may be a functional abnormality such as the rise of intra-ocular pressure in glaucoma or an anatomical abnormality such as the cysts in polycystic renal disease.

Unfortunately it is not possible always to define a disease on the basis of a precise and constant characteristic and then a polythetic concept of disease becomes useful. For example, the collagen diseases are a group of conditions in which there is considerable clinical, histological, and serological overlap and none has a defining feature present in every case of the one and absent from every case of the other. The non-specific inflammatory diseases of the colon also fall into this polythetic category.

NUMERICAL TAXONOMY
For the classification of polythetic diseases the technique of numerical taxonomy may be helpful. It involves comparing the characteristics of each patient with every other, the resemblance between any two patients being expressed numerically as a similarity coefficient. Clustering methods can then be used to group the coefficients so that the patients in a cluster resemble each other more than they resemble members of other clusters. There are various clustering techniques that can be used. Suffice it to say that most start with the two most similar patients as the initial members of the first cluster and the next patient to join is the one closest to either of the initial two. The cluster continues to be built up by the successive addition of single patients or groups of patients depending on the method, until none sufficiently close to the cluster can be found. That cluster is then complete and the next starts forming with the closest pair of patients not already in a cluster. When no sufficiently close pair is found the clustering process stops.

Perhaps it is worth emphasizing that numerical taxonomy makes no prior assumption as to whether or not the population studied is divisible into groups. Thus it is quite different from discriminant analysis which gives weight to the diagnostic features of two known groups.

APPLICATION OF NUMERICAL TAXONOMY TO MEDICINE
So far there has been little experience of the application of numerical taxonomy to medicine though it has been used very successfully with bacteria (Sneath, 1964). Using this technique, Hayhoe, Quaglino, and Doll (1966) were able to classify acute leukaemias on the basis of cytology and cytochemistry. Baron and Fraser (1968) applied numerical analysis to the classification of chronic liver disease using clinical as well as biochemical and

histological characters but encountered difficulties which may have been due in part to the retrospective nature of their data. Because of dissatisfaction with current psychiatric diagnostic schemes, Lorr (1966) employed clustering techniques for the classification of psychotic patients: the types identified in this way proved to be reliable in that there was good agreement between two independent raters in placing patients in these categories.

With the help of Professor Card, Professor Sneath, and Dr. Spicer we have been using clustering procedures as a new way of tackling the taxonomic problem of non-specific colitis.

APPLICATION OF NUMERICAL TAXONOMY TO NON-SPECIFIC COLITIS

The existence of proctocolitis (ulcerative colitis) has long been accepted but only in recent years has it been recognized that the inflammatory process first described by Crohn and his colleagues in the ileum may affect the colon without ileal involvement so providing another type of non-specific colitis (Wells, 1952; Lockhart-Mummery and Morson, 1964). This type has the same pathological features as the small bowel disease and has been termed 'Crohn's disease of the colon'. The features used for differentiating proctocolitis from colonic Crohn's disease have recently been reviewed by Lennard-Jones, Lockhart-Mummery, and Morson (1968). Although the two types of colitis differ in their clinical, radiological, and pathological characteristics neither has a defining feature present in every case of the one and absent from every case of the other. Thus this is a polythetic situation and patients with non-specific colitis are assigned to one or other group after an assessment of their overall similarity to the members of that group. The differential diagnosis is often extremely difficult and some workers consider that the two conditions overlap to such an extent that no clear separation can be made between them (Lewin and Swales, 1966; Thayer, 1967; Goldstein, Schachter, Rappaport, Fennessey, and Kirsner, 1968). It is not known whether there are two separate diseases which sometimes stimulate one another very closely or whether these types of colitis form opposite ends of a distribution curve representing a variety of reactions of the body to one aetiological agent.

The relationship between the two types of colitis will only finally be resolved when their aetiology is known. In the meantime we felt that an objective mathematical analysis of non-specific colitis might prove helpful by showing whether the disease patterns currently recognized separate out as distinct groups or whether they form a homogeneous group or whether a new classification might emerge.

The patients we studied by numerical taxonomy were a series of 109 patients with non-specific colitis, consecutively admitted to St. Mark's Hospital under Dr. Lennard-Jones's care. Those with previous colonic resections were excluded and so also were patients who did not have a barium enema or rectal biopsy examination. Of the 109 patients, 35 had a colectomy, and macroscopic and microscopic data from the operation specimen were included in the study.

A total of 156 attributes was chosen to represent features of the disease in each patient including data from the operation specimen. The attributes used were defined as carefully as possible, graded where appropriate, and coded in numerical form suitable for handling by a computer before being entered in a proforma. Clinical assessment of each patient included history, physical examination and sigmoidoscopy, and was represented by 54 attributes. Haematological and biochemical data included haemoglobin, E.S.R., liver-function tests, plasma proteins and immunoglobulin estimations (13 attributes). Pathological data, which was assessed with Dr. Morson, was obtained from rectal biopsy specimens (14 attributes) and from operation specimens (47 attributes) when the latter were available. Radiological attributes (26) were assessed from barium enema and small bowel films with Dr. Chapman. Age and sex accounted for a further two attributes.

From assessment of the clinical and radiological data, and the results of rectal biopsy, a clinical diagnosis of proctocolitis was made in 61 patients and of colonic Crohn's disease in 36 patients; it was not possible to distinguish between these two types of colitis in the remaining 12 patients. These clinical decisions were made before the data was analysed by the computer. The program used for the taxonomic analysis was Carmichael's TAXON and the data was run on the University of Leicester computer by M. J. Sackin.

The results of the computer output (*Fig.* 4) are expressed in a taxometric map (Carmichael and Sneath, 1969) in which differences between patients are represented by distance using a suitable scale. Though this is a convenient method for displaying relations between groups, an accurate simultaneous representation of all the distances between more than three points is not possible in a two-dimensional system. Thus a diagram of this kind inevitably involves some distortion though the main relationships are preserved. The circles represent clusters of patients sufficiently similar to one another and dissimilar from all other patients to be regarded as a distinct group. The diameter of each circle is dependent on the maximum difference between the patients in that group.

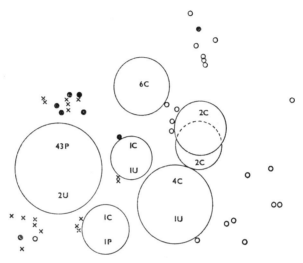

Fig. 4.—Taxometric map showing the results of cluster analysis of 109 patients with non-specific colitis using clinical, radiological, and pathological data. **x** = Proctocolitis. **O** = Crohn's. **●** = Uncertain. 0.1 sim unit = 1 inch.

Thus the fact that the diameter of the circle containing 45 patients is only slightly greater than that of the circle containing 5 patients indicates that the overall similarity of the patients in the larger cluster is greater than that of the smaller cluster. The distance between the circles depends on the overall difference between the groups.

The individual points represent single patients who were not sufficiently similar to the members of any group to be included in one. Most of the single points have some similarity to particular clusters and are termed 'satellites' of those clusters, but others are completely isolated.

Fig. 4 shows the results obtained when all the attributes were used in the analysis except those derived from the operation specimen, which was only available in about a third of the patients. There were 7 clusters in the computer output. The largest contained 45 patients, comprising 43 labelled clinically as 'proctocolitis' and 2 of uncertain diagnosis. The other 6 clusters were composed mainly of patients regarded as having colonic Crohn's disease, apart from 2 patients of uncertain diagnosis and 1 labelled as 'proctocolitis'. Scattered around the main cluster and some of the smaller clusters was a number of unclustered points, among which were over half the patients whom we had labelled as Crohn's disease.

It is apparent that this computer analysis of non-specific colitis has produced not an amorphous mixture of patients but separate clusters. One large cluster of patients corresponds fairly closely with a clinical diagnosis of proctocolitis and several smaller clusters correspond broadly with a clinical diagnosis of colonic Crohn's disease. Thus this spatial representation of patients with non-specific inflammatory disease of the colon supports the concept of separate disease groups. Moreover, it suggests that the disorder now termed 'proctocolitis' comprises a single, relatively uniform group of patients, whereas what is described as 'colonic Crohn's disease' is more heterogeneous and may be composed of distinguishable sub-groups.

ASSESSMENT OF DIFFERENT DIAGNOSTIC DISCIPLINES

The same technique was used to find how the patients cluster using just one type of attribute alone. Use of clinical data only (*Fig.* 5) produced a pattern of clusters similar to that obtained using all the data. There were 6 clusters. The largest contained 44 patients labelled as 'proctocolitis', 4 labelled as 'Crohn's disease' and 1 of uncertain diagnosis. One small cluster in close proximity to the main cluster contained a further 2 patients, diagnosed as proctocolitis. The remaining 4 clusters contained mainly patients labelled as 'Crohn's disease'. As in *Fig.* 4 there was a considerable number of unclustered points.

When the radiological data was analysed the picture was more complex (*Fig.* 6). There were 11 clusters. The largest contained 28 patients labelled as 'proctocolitis', 3 diagnosed as 'Crohn's disease' and 2 of uncertain diagnosis. Of the next two largest clusters, one contained 8 patients labelled as 'proctocolitis' and 3 labelled as 'Crohn's disease', and the other comprised 3 patients diagnosed as proctocolitis and 2 of uncertain diagnosis. Both these clusters and 5 smaller ones were in close proximity to the main group. The 3

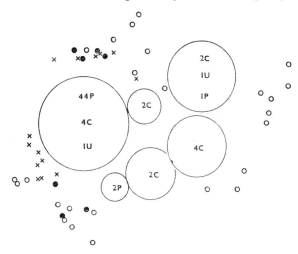

Fig. 5.—Taxometric map showing the results of cluster analysis of 109 patients with non-specific colitis using only clinical data. **x** = **Procto-colitis. O** = **Crohn's. ●** = **Uncertain.** o·1 sim unit = 1 inch.

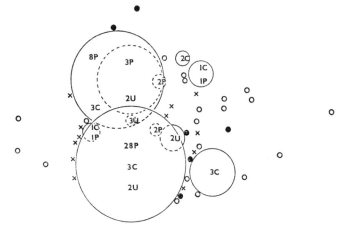

Fig. 6.—Taxometric map showing the results of cluster analysis of 109 patients with non-specific colitis using only radiological data. **x** = **Procto-colitis. O** = **Crohn's. ●** = **Uncertain.** o·1 sim unit = 1 inch.

remaining clusters lying on one side of the above groups contained mainly patients diagnosed as Crohn's disease. There was a considerable proportion of unclustered patients. Thus the correlation between the computer groups and the clinical diagnoses was less clear than in the previous analyses and the patients labelled clinically as 'proctocolitis' tended to fall into several clusters.

Analysis of the rectal biopsy data alone (*Fig.* 7) produced 8 clusters. The largest contained a total of 64 patients (over half the total number in the series) of whom 34 had been diagnosed clinically as proctocolitis, 23 as Crohn's disease and 7 were of uncertain diagnosis. Four small clusters contained only patients

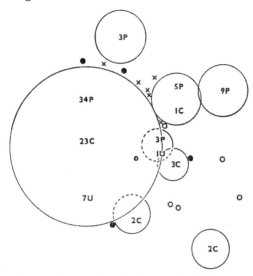

Fig. 7.—Taxometric map showing the results of cluster analysis of 109 patients with non-specific colitis using only data from rectal biopsy specimens. **x** = **Proctocolitis.** **O** = **Crohn's.** ● = **Uncertain.** 0.1 sim unit = 1 inch.

with proctocolitis apart from 1 patient diagnosed as having Crohn's disease and 1 of uncertain diagnosis. Three other small clusters contained only patients diagnosed as having Crohn's disease. These results suggested that there was poor computer discrimination between the clinical types of colitis on the basis of these histological criteria from the rectal biopsy.

Analysis of the macroscopic and microscopic data from the operation specimen produced 3 clusters (*Fig.* 8). The largest cluster contained 21 patients diagnosed as proctocolitis. Of the other 2 clusters, one contained 4 patients labelled as Crohn's disease, 1 labelled as proctocolitis and 3 of uncertain diagnosis; the other contained 2 patients diagnosed as Crohn's disease.

There were only 4 satellites—1 labelled as 'proctocolitis' and 3 as 'Crohn's disease'. Thus, unlike the rectal biopsy, the operation specimen provided sufficient data for a clear differentiation to be made between the clinical types of colitis in the limited number of patients who had a colectomy.

In this way numerical taxonomy has allowed an assessment of the relative value of the different disciplines used in the differential diagnosis of colonic inflammatory disease. The results suggest that the clinician's assessment of the patient including history, examination, and sigmoidoscopy is specially useful. Radiological data alone is less helpful. Histological criteria from rectal biopsy

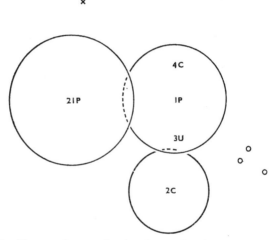

Fig. 8.—Taxometric map showing the results of cluster analysis of 35 patients with non-specific colitis using only data from the operation specimen. **x** = **P**roctocolitis. **O** = **C**rohn's. ● = **U**ncertain. 0·1 sim unit = 1 inch.

examinations give relatively poor discrimination but data from operation specimens, when these are available, correlates well with the clinical diagnoses.

ANALYSIS USING DISCRIMINANT ATTRIBUTES ONLY

Returning to the picture produced by analysis of all the attributes, it is apparent that the smaller clusters all fell on one side of the main cluster, and it was possible to divide the patients into two groups which we labelled A and B.

Group A comprised the main cluster and its satellites and consisted mainly of patients diagnosed as proctocolitis; and group B comprised the other clusters and their satellites and consisted largely of patients labelled as 'colonic Crohn's disease'.

To determine which attributes contributed most to this separation, the mean value of each attribute was calculated in these two groups, A and B, and the '*t*' test was used to pick out those attributes in which the means differed significantly in the two groups. The computer analysis was then repeated using only these attributes (47 in number) to test the effect of eliminating unhelpful characters on the clustering process.

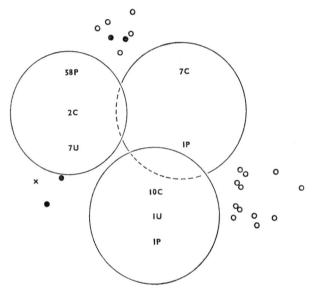

Fig. 9.—Taxometric map showing the results of cluster analysis of 109 patients with non-specific colitis using only discriminant attributes. x = **Proctocolitis.** O = **Crohn's.** ● = **Uncertain.** o·1 sim unit = 1 inch.

The results are shown in *Fig.* 9. Three clusters were produced. The largest contained all the patients diagnosed as proctocolitis, except 3. The other two clusters contained mainly patients diagnosed as Crohn's disease, though there were still a considerable number of patients with this clinical label who were similar to, but not included in, these two clusters. Compared with the previous analysis using all 109 characters, it is evident that using these 47 characters has produced fewer clusters containing more patients, but the heterogeneity of the disorder known as 'colonic Crohn's disease' is still manifest. This suggests that elimination of 'noise' or unhelpful characters may help to clarify the taxonomic picture while the basic pattern is preserved.

LIMITATIONS AND POSSIBILITIES OF NUMERICAL TAXONOMY

Claims that numerical taxonomy makes classification objective are only partly true. In the first place, the choice of attributes or characters is still subjective though the degree of subjectivity can be reduced by using a large number of attributes representing all aspects of the disease process. Secondly, the choice of patients is also subjective as in any clinical study though this is mitigated by study of a consecutive series of patient admissions to hospital. Thirdly, the accuracy of the data is open to criticism especially when dealing with symptoms. Many patients differ in what they mean when they use such common words as diarrhoea, pain, flatulence, or arthritis and it is therefore mandatory for the investigator to use vocabulary which is quite unambiguous (Boyle, 1970). Even with a questionnaire of fixed format such as we have used in the present study, different patients may interpret the same wording differently so that the impression of standardization of data conveyed by a proforma may be misleading.

There is some degree of arbitrariness in the technique of cluster analysis itself. The computer groups patients together according to their degree of similarity and the criteria for formation of a group or cluster are defined by the program. Since a variety of clustering techniques are available and since each technique has its own criteria for the definition of a cluster, the results will depend to some extent on the particular technique employed. This has been demonstrated by Wishart (1969) who used various methods of cluster analysis to test 30 characters elicited from a number of patients each of whom was known to have one of three types of non-toxic goitre. He found that the results of 8 methods ranged from complete failure to almost complete success in obtaining groups which correlated with the clinical diagnoses. Such variation in results with different techniques suggests that the results of a particular cluster analysis should not be accepted unless the clusters make sense in terms of the biological or medical field involved. Moreover, it is important that any taxonomic program should be justified by demonstrating that it can reproduce a known configuration of units, given the necessary data, before it is used in biological or medical projects. We chose Carmichael's program because it was convenient to do so and because it had been validated in a test system (Carmichael and Sneath, 1969).

At present there is no statistical means of predicting the probability of a distribution being single or bimodal and with a multimodal distribution the problem is even more complex (Moran, 1969). Thus the likelihood of the results of cluster analysis occurring by chance alone cannot be assessed. It follows that numerical taxonomy is essentially a descriptive rather than a statistical technique. The problem is made more complex by the recent demonstration by Day (1969), that apparent bimodality of a pronounced degree occurs in random samples from a multivariate normal population to a far greater extent than one might expect.

Even if clusters could be identified with certainty, their significance in the analysis of a disease state may be uncertain. This is because the same disease can affect different anatomical systems, as in tuberculosis, may manifest itself in different immunological forms, as in the lepromatous and tuberculoid forms of leprosy, or can produce two quite different groups of symptoms at different times as in manic-depressive psychosis. We do not know how far apart the clusters must be to justify the label of different diseases.

We are only just beginning to feel our way with numerical taxonomy in medicine so that at present one can only speculate on the ways in which it might prove useful in the future. It may have a place in the classification of disease groups of unknown aetiology which are defined in a polythetic manner. By providing a classification which may include new groups numerical taxonomy could stimulate ideas about the aetiology of the groups it identifies. When the classification is based on a mass of information derived from many variables in a large number of patients the analysis would obviously be difficult without a computer.

It is possible that the biggest potential of the technique lies in treatment and prognosis rather than in classification. Within any one disease patients may vary greatly depending on the presence or absence of features which influence prognosis. Goldstein and Mackay (1967) at Melbourne have demonstrated how computer techniques can be used to identify subsets of patients which can be linked with a particular treatment. They correlated histological, clinical, biochemical, and serological findings at various stages in 30 patients with lupoid hepatitis and were able to define a 'hepatitis phase' characterized by liver cell necrosis and a 'cirrhosis phase' characterized by fibrosis and loss of architecture. They found that liver cell necrosis correlated inversely with corticosteroid dosage and thus showed that the hepatitis phase was improved by corticosteroid treatment. In this way computer programs can be geared to therapy rather than to classification alone.

Numerical taxonomy might be of interest for studying the progression of a disease by demonstrating a changing pattern of clusters with passage of time. For example, if a given population of patients formed one large cluster at the first analysis but several clusters at a later date, the implication would be that there was a disorder of single aetiology which later developed diverse manifestations under the influence of environmental or other factors. Alternatively, analysis at an early date might produce several clusters which subsequently merged to form one, suggesting the existence of separate disorders which ultimately developed a close resemblance.

CONCLUSION

In conclusion, I have outlined the concept of numerical taxonomy and discussed its application to colonic inflammatory disease. The computer results largely support clinical impressions about the classification of nonspecific colitis and perhaps this is not surprising since the human mind is very good at taxonomy. We have applied a new mathematical technique to a current clinical problem and we hope that our experience in doing so may stimulate people into thinking about other fields in which the technique might be useful.

REFERENCES

BARON, D. N., and FRASER, P. M. (1968), 'Medical Applications of Taxonomic Methods', Br. med. Bull., 24, 236.

BOYLE, C. H. (1970), 'Difference between Patients' and Doctors' Interpretation of some Common Medical Terms', Br. med. J., 2, 286.

CARMICHAEL, J. W., and SNEATH, P. H. A. (1969), 'Taxometric Maps', Syst. Zool., 18, 402.

DAY, N. E. (1969), 'Estimating the Components of a Mixture of Normal Distributions', Biometrika, 56, 3, 463.

GOLDSTEIN, G., and MACKAY, I. R. (1967), 'Lupoid Hepatitis: Computer Analysis defining "Hepatitis" and "Cirrhosis" Phases and Relationships between Hepatocellular Damage and Immune Reactions in the Liver', Australas. Ann. Med., 16, 62.

GOLDSTEIN, M. J., SCHACHTER, H., RAPPAPORT, H., FENNESSEY, J. J., and KIRSNER, J. B. (1968), 'Ulcerative and Granulomatous Colitis—Validity of Differential Criteria: A Study of 100 Patients treated by Total Colectomy', Gastroenterology, 54, 1241.

J. HYWEL JONES

HAYHOE, F. G. J., QUAGLINO, D., and DOLL, W. R. S. (1966) 'The Cytology and Cytochemistry of Acute Leukaemias'. *Spec. Rep. Ser. Med. Res. Coun.*, No. 304. London: H.M.S.O

LENNARD-JONES, J. E., LOCKHART-MUMMERY, H. E., and MORSON, B. C. (1968), 'Clinical and Pathological Differentiation of Crohn's Disease and Proctocolitis', *Gasteroenterology*, **54,** 1162.

LEWIN, K., and SWALES, J. D. (1966), 'Granulomatous Colitis and Atypical Ulcerative Colitis. Histological Features, Behaviour and Prognosis', *Ibid.*, **50,** 211.

LOCKHART-MUMMERY, H. E., and MORSON, B. C. (1964), 'Crohn's Disease of the Large Intestine', *Gut*, **5,** 493.

LORR, M. (ed.), (1966), *Exploration in Typing Psychotics*. Oxford: Pergamon.

MORAN, P. A. P. (1969), 'Statistical Methods in Psychiatric Research', *Jl R. statist. Soc.*, **132,** 484.

SCADDING, J. G. (1967), 'Diagnosis: the Clinician and the Computer', *Lancet*, **2,** 877.

SNEATH, P. H. A. (1962), 'The Construction of Taxonomic Groups'. In *Microbial Classification*, 12th Symposium Soc. gen. Microbiol. (ed. AINSWORTH' G. C., and SNEATH, P. H. A.). p. 289. London: Cambridge University Press.

— — (1964), 'New Approaches to Bacterial Taxonomy. Use of Computers', *A. Rev. Microbiol.*, **18,** 335.

SOKAL, R. R., and SNEATH, P. H. A. (1963), *Principles of Numerical Taxonomy*. San Francisco: Freeman.

THAYER, W. R. (1967), 'Comment on Article by B. I. Korelitz', *Gastroenterology*, **53,** 998.

WELLS, C. (1952), 'Ulcerative Colitis and Crohn's Disease', *Ann. R. Coll. Surg. Engl.*, **11,** 105.

WISHART, D. (1969), 'The Use of Cluster Analysis in the Classification of Diseases', *Scott. med. J.*, **14,** 96.

DISCUSSION

Comment (Professor Scadding): I will claim a chairman's privilege and make two observations before asking for questions and discussion on Dr. Jones' paper.

First, it is interesting that attempts to apply computers to medical diagnosis have demonstrated the continuing importance of the mediaeval controversy between nominalists and realists on the nature of universals. Implicitly, if not explicitly, the notion of cluster analysis is based upon a realist view of 'diseases'. Numerical taxonomy is applicable to material objects, like plants, insects, and bacteria, that can be dissected and analysed to yield features by which they can be identified; and the application of this technique to diseases would be appropriate only if they are, or can be regarded as, real entities. But I think that the general concept 'a disease' can be analysed intelligibly only on uncompromisingly nominalist principles, in the tradition of British empirical philosophers from Locke, Berkeley, and Hume to Russell. It is true that the names of diseases are used in medical discourse as if they referred to agents causing symptoms and signs in a patient, and the grammatical structure of Western languages encourages this naïve supposition. But only if knowledge were so complete that the cause of every illness could be

73

discovered, so that each could be classified with others having the same cause, and all diseases were therefore definable in terms of causes—i.e., aetiologically—would this viewpoint be plausible, and even then only with important reservations. In practice, and inevitably in the present state of medical knowledge, the diagnostic process more often than not stops short of its desirable end-point, causation. We may be able to carry it no further than recognition of a combination of clinical symptoms and signs, in which event we classify the patient with others presenting a similar clinical picture. If abnormalities of structure of function can be demonstrated, they may constitute a more useful criterion, and therefore tend to displace the symptom-complex as basis of classification. When causes of disease are recognized, diagnostic categories based on aetiology usually displace all others.

We thus have a number of different sorts of criterion for definition of diagnostic categories. The concept 'a disease' is a convenient logical device by which we can refer to the sum of the abnormal phenomena observed in patients falling into one of these diagnostic categories. This analysis admits the logical heterogeneity of 'diseases' and is an essential preliminary to any discussion of the application of computers to diagnosis. Such discussion is hopelessly confused as long as it is conducted in terms of 'diseases' regarded uncritically as a logically homogeneous group of agents causing these symptoms. But once we accept the view that when we use the name of a disease we are simply referring to all the phenomena we observe in a group of patients defined by the possession of a common characteristic, and that this common defining characteristic may belong to any one of several different fields of study, we will not be surprised to find that all the more successful applications of computers to medical diagnosis have been concerned with groups of cases belonging to diagnostic categories having defining characteristics in a single field of study (Scadding, 1967).

Secondly, I would draw attention to Dr. Jones' comment that there is no objective criterion of the 'correctness' of cluster analysis. It seems to me that unless a group of cases identified by this technique can be shown to have a common characteristic which makes possible its definition on the basis of morbid anatomy, aetiology, or one of the other accepted criteria of diagnostic categorization, the delineation of groups detectable only by computer analysis is likely to obscure rather than clarify nosology.

REFERENCE

Scadding, J. G. (1967), 'Diagnosis: the Clinician and the Computer', Lancet, 2, 877.

Comment (Professor B. Lennox): May I make two points, one theoretical and one practical?

The theoretical one is this: I don't think that there exists such a thing as a monothetic human disease. Take Dr. Jones' example of tuberculosis. On the one hand, one often has to accept the diagnosis of tuberculosis without being able to demonstrate the tubercle bacillus. Of course, one assumes the bacillus is there and it probably is, but one cannot both accept the assumption and accept the presence as necessary to the diagnosis. On the other hand, the tubercle bacillus is not the only diagnostic factor. If the tubercle bacillus was not accompanied by other signs significantly more often than for normal individuals, if it was the sole distinguishing feature between a case of tuberculosis and a normal person, then tuberculosis would not be a disease.

Comment (Professor J. G. Scadding): At first glance, and without wishing to commit myself without further consideration, I wonder whether it may not be possible to correlate the notion of monothetic and polythetic categorization of disease with my analysis of the concept 'a disease'. My present impression is that those diseases that are defined in terms of a specified causal factor could be regarded as monothetic: those in terms of a specified disorder of function or a specified anatomical abnormality in most instances as monothetic; and those definable only on a clinical-descriptive basis as polythetic. But whether this distinction adds anything useful to my analysis, I do not know.

Professor B. Lennox (continues): I don't think we ought to become involved too much in the discussion of this. I only wanted to make sure that some innocent computer men in the audience might not go away with the idea that monothetic and polythetic groups were a matter of indisputable doctrine!

The practical matter is this: Dr. Jones showed a table in which sarcoid granulomata were recorded in no cases of ulcerative colitis and in 60 per cent of cases of Crohn's disease. If this is so, why was cluster analysis of the pathological findings unable to give any clear distinction between them?

Answer: The frequency of granulomas I gave in the table represented Dr. Morson's findings in his previous work on operation specimens from patients with the different types of colitis. When we used data from colectomy specimens in the present study we did in fact get a good correlation with the clinical diagnoses though relatively few patients diagnosed as Crohn's disease came to surgery. The clustering was poor only when we used the limited data from the rectal biopsies and in these the incidence of granulomas was very small.

Professor B. Lennox: I see. If the table applied to resection cases only and the analysis to biopsy cases only, the discrepancy is easy to understand.

PANEL DISCUSSION*
(Professor Anderson, Professor Donaldson)

Question (Dr. A. W. Cull): What about basic decision making?

Answer (Professor J. Anderson): The system at King's College Hospital Medical School has been programmed to be able to make decisions

---

* At the end of the first day's proceedings.

at a very low level about orders and responses. Programs exist for surveying data but do not make decisions as a result of this analysis. So far we have not explored diagnostic decision making.

Question (Dr. C. R. Hearn): How do you start this process ?

Answer (Professor J. Anderson): This is done by discussion with all concerned to see what is acceptable and what errors can be tolerated if made by programs. All systems must be thoroughly tested in a test bed area before general implementation.

Question (Dr. O. C. Parry-Jones): How do you tackle difficulties concerning the provision of summaries for various interested parties ?

Answer (Professor J. Anderson): Users find it difficult to specify what they want. Usually people think they want all the information and are only educated when they see a mass of print-out. They tend to take data reduction for granted. Different users have different requirements for summaries. Thus, doctors and G.Ps. want a medical summary, while nurses or administrators want a different type of summary dealing with activities.

Question (Dr. K. T. Gruer): If your system were to be adopted generally, some difficulties would arise. It would be important to provide suitable tuition to medical students in order to make the system work. Is this being done ?

Answer (Professor J. Anderson): We are already teaching our students and nurses how to use the system and have been doing this for three years. It is evident that nurses are very keen to apply their knowledge, since the procedure saves time. Student teaching is now being expanded to include optional courses in elementary programming and system analysis.

A question: Have you investigated patient questionnaires ?

Answer (Professor J. Anderson): We are giving patient questionnaires to G.P.s who give them to the patients they send to us. The patients will then fill them in and post these to the hospital, where they are punched-up and a print-out is available for the doctor at the out-patient consultation. This saves a great deal of work and time, and much more information is available.

Question (Professor F. W. Donaldson): Is there a formal curriculum available in this field to medical students ?

Answer (Professor J. Anderson): There is no formal curriculum, only a timetable as yet has been approved by the Academic Board.

Question (B. Day): You mentioned that it would take 10 years to fully implement a total system. If such a real-time system is cost effective, then the sooner the whole system can be implemented the greater will be the resultant savings. Is there any inherent reason why such a hospital information system should require three times the time-scale of a comparable commercial system ?

Answer (Professor J. Anderson): Commercial systems may also take 10 years to be fully implemented such as the BEA system. It is not possible to implement complete hospital systems in much less time, allowing for education of users and the various changes in attitudes and types of work. Also there are very few managers in the business who in fact could implement a total system on the experimental data we have available so far.

Question (B. Day): Would it not be possible to reduce this long preparatory time by bringing in consultants, suppliers, and others at the beginning of the exercise?

Answer (Professor J. Anderson): It is not easy to convince consultants and others quickly; an interactive process is essential. Some speed-up may be possible by building up real-time systems quickly and getting communications underway using suitable computers. Nevertheless the investment in computers for the whole of the health service is bound to be large and adequate experiments must proceed before full implementation. In fact, some stimulation studies are being done now.

Question (D. D. Rose): Our experience is that systems involving satellites can be established very quickly.

Answer (Professor J. Anderson): To see is to believe.

Question (J. R. Brooke): Would Professor Anderson, please, give an estimate of costs, time, etc., of this system?

Answer (Professor J. Anderson): I cannot answer this question in detail as the experiments are not yet concluded. Costs depend on hardware, and programming methods used. There are also difficulties in transferring software from one manufacturers computer to another. We are also having some design difficulties as users find established procedures changing and so want new ones created. In a dynamic system like this it is difficult to quote costs in the long run.

Question (D. D. Rose): How many doctors serve the poor area of Memphis, what is the size of the actual area and what computer facilities exist?

Answer (Professor F. W. Donaldson): The area involved is 10 miles long and 5 miles wide with a population of 50,000 people. Within this area (15–20 miles radius from Memphis) there are a few small hospitals and about 100 doctors (full-time and part-time). The computer is an I.B.M. 360/40 plus. This is inadequate for our needs and will have to be upgraded. It is hoped to locate the equipment in preventive medicine centres and out-patient clinics, as well as to provide multiphasic screening at centres. The time required for the system becoming fully operational, as described in the lecture, is about 6 months.

Question (Dr. A. Fernandez): What is the cost of the E.C.G. interpretation system in Memphis?

Answer (Professor F. W. Donaldson): One E.C.G. interpretation by computer costs about $2. About 4000 interpretations are done daily. As regards hardware, the cost of the 1700 system used for E.C.G. interpretation is about $200,000. The central facility, by the way, consists of 2 magnetic tapes, 1 disk file, memory of 106 bytes, teleprinters, and ancillary equipment.

77

SESSION 3

Chairman: Dr. J. H. Mitchell

The learn'd is happy nature to explore.
The fool is happy that he knows no more.

ALEXANDER POPE

Electrocardiographic potential mapping by computer

B. D. Young and T. D. V. Lawrie

ELECTROCARDIOGRAPHY is concerned with the measurement and interpretation of the electrical signals generated by the heart. The systems in current clinical use, viz., the conventional 12-lead system and the 3-lead vectorcardiographic systems, record electrocardiograms (E.C.G.s) from electrodes placed on the limbs and the thorax. Electrocardiographic potential mapping which displays the activity of the entire thorax surface has been developed to investigate whether significant information is available at areas not examined by conventional lead systems. This technique involves recording E.C.G.s sequentially from a large number of points on the thorax and combining these signals into a series of instantaneous isopotential contour maps throughout the cardiac cycle. To provide accurate time correlation a limb lead is recorded simultaneously with each thoracic signal. Thus in contrast to conventional techniques the sequence of electrical activity produced by the heart can be observed over the entire thorax.

The first isopotential study of the human body was by Nahum, Mauro, Chernoff, and Sickland (1951) who produced two maps during the QRS complex of the electrocardiogram (i.e., during ventricular depolarization). This early work was developed further by Taccardi (1963, 1966) who derived a greater number of maps from the QRS complex, the P wave (atrial depolarization) and the T wave (ventricular repolarization). The most significant technical advance in this field has been the introduction of digital

78

computers to handle the large amounts of data involved. Horan, Flowers, and Brody (1963) and Spach and others (1966) developed computer techniques for plotting isopotential contours from E.C.G. waveforms recorded on analogue magnetic tape. After a preliminary study by the author (Young, 1967) a method has been developed in this laboratory whereby thoracic E.C.G.s are recorded directly from the patient by computer and the results plotted automatically as a series of isopotential contour maps. This technique is currently being used in a study of the thoracic activity of both normal patients and those known to have ischaemic heart disease.

ACQUISITION OF DATA

The data acquisition system is shown diagrammatically in *Fig.* 10. Electrocardiographic amplifiers linked the patient's body on-line to a PDP-8 computer which included 8K of 12-bit core store,

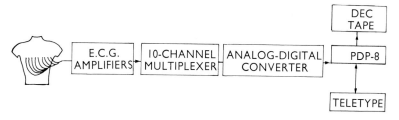

Fig. 10.—Data acquisition by PDP-8 computer.

2 digital magnetic tape units, a 10-channel multiplexer and analog-digital converter, and an 80-column line printer. The E.C.G. amplifiers were constructed from integrated micro-circuit amplifiers to produce 9 chest E.C.G.s with the Wilson Central Terminal as their voltage reference and limb Lead II as a common time reference. Typical output signals are shown in *Fig.* 11 in which the chest E.C.G.s numbered from 1 to 9, correspond to electrode positions from right to left on the thorax.

The PDP-8 was programmed to process and store 9 simultaneous Q–T intervals on digital magnetic tape. The effects of respiration were minimized by recording data at a fixed point in the respiration cycle. On completion of this operation the thoracic electrodes were moved to a new position and the data acquisition program was run 14 times until signals from 126 points had been processed. In this way Q–T intervals were obtained from a

7 × 18 array of sites covering most of the thorax, the whole procedure requiring about 45 minutes for one patient.

DATA ACQUISITION PROGRAM

The acquisition and storage of E.C.G. waveforms were controlled by a computer program written in PAL, the PDP-8 assembly language. Communication with this program was via

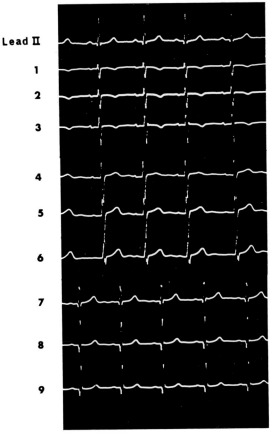

Fig. 11.—Output signals from E.C.G. amplifiers.

the computer teletype. Before an analog waveform, such as an electrocardiogram, can be handled by a digital computer it must be converted into a sequence of amplitude measurements. This process, known as 'digitization', took place at a rate of 500 samples per sec. on each channel with a resolution of 12 bits ($\pm$0·025 per cent), in accordance with the recommendations of the American Heart Association (1967). Prior to each conversion the multi-plexer, a high-speed electronic switch, connected the appropriate E.C.G. signal to the analog-digital converter. Although the ideal technique would have been simultaneous digitization on all input channels, the multiplexer provided such rapid switching that sequential sampling was satisfactory. The time required for each 12-bit conversion was 35 μsec.

The first part of the program calibrated the amplifiers by measuring the amplitude of ten 1 mV. square wave signals on each of the nine chest leads. The maximum, minimum, and mean of these values were printed and, if acceptable, the program continued with the mean values taken as scaling factors for all subsequent E.C.G. data.

The calibration signal was also used to initiate the signal processing and therefore it was necessary to develop a programme technique to differentiate between that waveform and the relatively large R wave of the QRS complex. By finding the difference (ΔV) between two successive values from the analog-digital converter for a given channel, the 1 mV. calibration and R wave signals were distinguished as follows:

$$UP < \Delta V \qquad \Rightarrow \text{Calibration signal}$$
$$LOW < \Delta V < UP \qquad \Rightarrow \text{R wave}$$

where UP and LOW are two constants whose values were set in advance. This method, which in effect measures the signal gradient, relies on the fact that the upstroke of the calibration is steeper than the R wave. Since, in practice, this was always the case, this simple approach provided reliable waveform detection.

The signal processing part of the program was designed to record digitally the Q–T interval of ten simultaneous E.C.G.s. However, because of the limited core store (4K) available for data storage, the high digitization rate (500 per sec.) and the relatively large number of simultaneous inputs, several data-handling problems had to be solved. For example, allocating 4K of core store equally between 10 channels with a sampling rate of 500 per sec. allows only 0·8 sec. of digitization. Hence with a heart-rate of 60 beats per sec. it would be possible to store only 80 per cent of the complete heart cycle, and this must include the Q–T interval. A further problem was that each of the sets of 9 chest E.C.G.s had to be alined with the peak of the R wave in limb Lead II as a common time reference.

81

These difficulties have been resolved by developing a technique of 'real time' detection of the limb lead R waves in such a way that they directly controlled the digitization procedures. A 'moving window' method of storage was adopted to allow the greatest flexibility in data handling. As each sample was obtained from the analog-digital converter it displaced a sample at the end of the appropriate 'window' and therefore a constant number of measurements was retained in a fixed area of core store. The leading edges of the 10 'windows', which were 0·8 sec. in length, thus always corresponded to real time.

The diagram in *Fig.* 12 illustrates in detail how the R waves of Lead II controlled digitization. The operator, having checked the

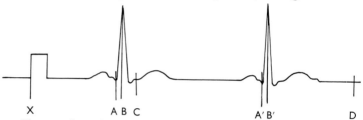

X   A B C   A′ B′   D

Fig. 12.—Control of digitization by R wave in limb Lead II. X, detect 1 mV. calibration and start search for R wave; A, detect R wave; B, detect peak of R wave; C, start to fill all data 'windows'; A′, detect R wave; B′, detect peak and continue sampling; D, stop sampling.

10 E.C.G. signals on a monitoring oscilloscope for excessive noise or baseline drift, initiated digitization with a calibration signal. This waveform was detected (point X in *Fig.* 12) using the criterion discussed earlier and hence, if the parameters LOW and UP were set correctly, it could not be confused with the QRS complex.

The next step was to wait for the R wave in Lead II and once this had been found (point A in *Fig.* 12) there was a short delay to allow the QRS complex to finish, followed by sampling on all channels to fill up the 'moving windows'. The program then continued by updating the 'windows' while waiting for the next R wave. After its detection (point A′ in *Fig.* 12) sampling continued for a further 0·508 sec. so that the final 'windows' included the Q–T interval of all 10 channels. As the peak of the R wave in Lead II had already been found all chest leads were correctly alined in time.

Certain calculations were carried out on the stored data. The baseline of each E.C.G. was found as the mean of 10 consecutive values (i.e., 0·02 sec.) at a point 0·128 sec. before the R wave peak of Lead II. The RMS deviations of these 10 points from their means were found and, if they exceeded a specified level, the appropriate channel number was printed. Thus it was possible to reject exceptionally noisy recordings and repeat the procedure while the electrodes were still in place. Likewise, the QRS complex of Lead II was also examined to ensure that no notching in the R wave had occurred since this could be mistaken for the peak.

Each stored E.C.G. was multiplied by its scaling factor, determined in the earlier part of the program. The scaled waveforms were printed on the teletype in a graphical form and by comparison with the original signals it was possible to decide whether correct digitization had taken place. If the data were satisfactory the nine thoracic E.C.G.s were transferred to digital magnetic tape for permanent storage, each channel being allocated 256 words which was equivalent to approximately 0·5 sec. The Lead II data, having served its purpose as a common time reference, was not stored.

The chest electrodes were then moved to a new position and the digitization process was restarted with another calibration signal. This was repeated until Q–T intervals from 14 sets of 9 electrode sites had been obtained.

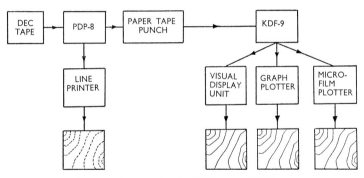

Fig. 13.—Isopotential mapping by PDP-8 and KDF9 computers.

DISPLAY OF THORACIC ACTIVITY

The most comprehensive presentation of the E.C.G. data is as a sequence of isopotential contour maps over the thorax. This approach was simplified by considering the thoracic surface as being 'unrolled' into a plane rectangle, the chest electrode sites thus taking the form of a 7×18 rectangular grid of points. The data for each contour map, which consisted of a set of 126 simultaneous potential measurements at each electrode, were compiled from the digital waveforms stored on magnetic tape. Mapping procedures which involved the interpolation and plotting of contour lines from this data, have been developed on both PDP-8 and KDF9 computers as illustrated in *Fig.* 13 and the principles of both techniques are discussed below.

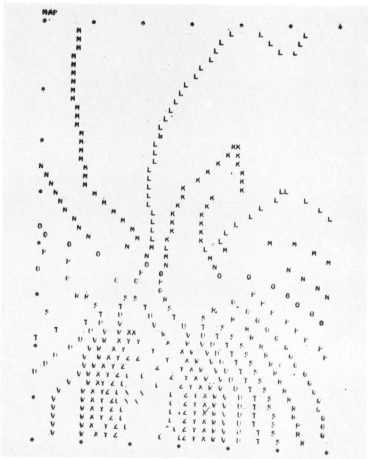

Fig. 14.—Isopotential map printed by PDP-8 in 'line' form.

ISOPOTENTIAL MAPPING BY PDP-8 COMPUTER

Since the PDP-8 computer did not include graph-plotting facilities a technique was devised to display potential distributions on the line printer or on a teletype. It was possible to produce maps in two different forms. As illustrated in *Fig.* 14 a particular alphabetic character could be used to plot the path of each contour line. Alternatively, characters could be used to mark areas between contours (*Fig.* 15) in which case the paths of contour lines

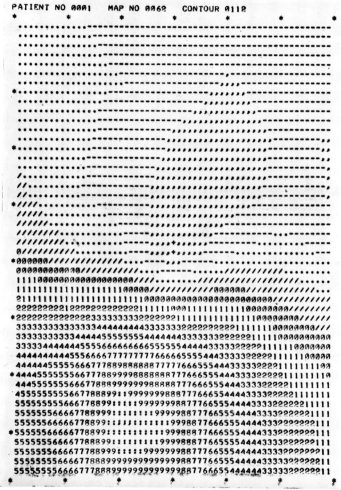

Fig. 15.—Isopotential map printed by PDP-8 in 'solid' form.

are indicated by the boundaries between different characters. Both illustrations correspond to a grid of 7 × 9 points, i.e., exactly half the total area examined.

In the first form the character 'o' denoted the zero isopotential (i.e., Wilson Central Terminal voltage) and in the second form the same character indicated areas of potential between zero and the first positive contour level. The interval between contours was selected according to the magnitude of the data, the most commonly used being 0·25 mV. (as in *Figs.* 14 and 15).

The principle of the interpolation procedure (Horan, Flowers, and Brody, 1963) was to subdivide each map into small regions, containing an equal number of data points, to which a potential surface was fitted in the following way. By considering each region to be m points in width and n points in length and using polynomial interpolation, the fitted surface for each area took the form:—

$$V(x, y) = (a_0 + a_1x + a_2x^2 + \ldots a_{n-1}x^{n-1})$$
$$X(b_0 + b_1y + b_2y^2 + \ldots b_{m-1}y^{m-1})$$

where $V(x, y)$ is potential at the point (x, y) and a_i ($i = 0,1 \ldots$, n–1) and b_j ($j = 0,1 \ldots$, m–1) are constant coefficients. It is evident from this equation that fitting such a surface required that k coefficients of the type a_ib_j be evaluated, where k is the product of m and n. This was accomplished by inserting the known values of V, x, and y into the above equation and solving the kth rank system of simultaneous linear equations thus obtained.

For routine purposes, the interpolation procedure was limited to its simplest form by processing the data in 2 × 2 blocks of points. Thus the potential equation reduced to:—

$$V(x, y) = ax + by + cxy + d$$

where a, b, c, and d are constants which can be evaluated from the potential data. This first order interpolation method was used to produce the maps in *Figs.* 14 and 15 and although it does not result in perfectly smooth contours it does give a satisfactory representation. Smoother isopotentials could have been obtained by use of a higher order interpolation with a larger data block (e.g., 3 × 3). However, the extra computing time required outweighed such possible improvements in the appearance of the maps.

Isopotential Mapping by KDF9 Computer

A mapping programme has been written in FORTRAN under the EGDON system of Glasgow University KDF9 computer to allow access to more sophisticated plotting facilities. This included a Calcomp incremental plotter, a visual display unit, and a micro-film plotter.

Although this approach had the disadvantage that data had to be reproduced as paper tape for transfer to the KDF9 computer, it provided accurate and conveniently annotated maps, one of which is illustrated in *Fig.* 16. This map was plotted from the same data as the map in *Fig.* 14; the contour levels, indicated at the edges of the map, are also the same. Simple interpolation was used whereby each isopotential was composed of straight line segments joining

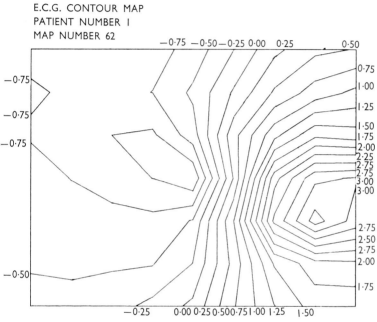

Fig. 16.—Isopotential map plotted by KDF9.

points of equal voltage. Although this resulted in sharp 'corners' to some of the contours, the consequent reduction in expensive computer time more than compensated any loss of definition.

The microfilm plotter, which is part of the KDF9 system at U.K.A.E.A. Culham Laboratories, has been used to produce a 16-mm. cine film of the changing distributions of thoracic potentials during the Q–T interval. This moving type of display, which is identical in form to the map in *Fig.* 16, illustrates clearly the sequence of electrocardiographic events which occur on the thorax.

Since the graphical output system of the KDF9 is independent of the plotting device the same mapping program was used to produce both the stationary maps and the cine film. However, the timing of the moving display had to be considered carefully. The digitization rate used by the data acquisition programme was 500 samples per sec. and hence the time between each map was 2 msec. If the maps for the QRS period (approximately 40) were printed by the microfilm plotter as sequential frames, then at a projection rate of 1500 frames per min. the display would last only 1·5 sec. It was therefore necessary to 'slow down' the display so that the events could be clearly observed. This could have been done by printing several frames of each map but the resulting movement of the isopotentials would have been rather spasmodic. However, by plotting several intermediate frames which merged linearly from one map to the next it was possible to obtain a display in which the contours appeared to move smoothly about the thorax. If the data for two original maps (2 msec. apart) are represented by the matrices P(t) and P(t + 1) and if the period between the maps is divided into s equal time intervals, then for each of the s

instants a map, represented by the matrix $P(t + \frac{r}{s})$ $(r = 0, 1, \dots$

s — 1), can be derived from P(t) and P(t + 1) by the definition:—

$$P(t + \frac{r}{s}) = P(t) + \frac{r}{s}(P(t + 1) - P(t)).$$

The first map is simply P(t) and the following maps approach P(t + 1) linearly. The plotting procedure consisted of printing such a set of s intermediate frames for each pair of maps. In practice the value of s used was 6 which, at a projection speed of 1500 frames per min., slowed down the display of the QRS period to approximately 9 sec.

DISCUSSION
Each of the four methods of producing maps (PDP-8 line printer, KDF9 graph plotter, visual display unit, and cine film) has certain advantages. The cine film technique clearly displays the relative motion of the potential maxima and minima over the thorax, a feature which is difficult to assess from a series of stationary maps. However, the production of such films is costly and time consuming and therefore at present is likely to be applied

to only a small number of patients. Although it is not possible to use the KDF9 visual display unit to produce an animated display it allows rapid inspection of a large number of maps in the form shown in *Fig.* 16. The graph plotter can also be used to provide a copy of such maps. This approach is at present limited by the transfer of data from the PDP-8 computer to the KDF9.

Use of the PDP-8 line printer, which involves no data transfer, is the most convenient, though least sophisticated method of mapping. Approximately 10 maps per min. can be produced in this way, the limiting factor being the calculation of isopotentials and not the speed of printing. The activity during the Q–T interval is presented as a sequence of 40 maps for each patient with contour levels of 0·25 mV. for the QRS period and 0·1 mV. for the T wave. Since these maps are compiled from E.C.G. waveforms recorded from 14 different cardiac cycles, the beat-to-beat variations of the surface potentials are assumed to be negligible. This has been justified by the agreement obtained between maps recorded on separate occasions.

Isopotential mapping was originally developed to investigate the accuracy of the single dipole model of the heart on which 12-lead electrocardiography and 3-lead vectorcardiography are based. Since then the technique has been used in the development of more sophisticated models. In this laboratory, work is in progress on the interpretation of contour maps using a multiple dipole model from which 'electrocardiograms' for discrete regions of the myocardium can be obtained.

Although it is now more than 20 years since the first isopotential study of the human thorax there is still a need for technical improvements before this branch of electrocardiography can be used routinely. The numbers of patients that can be studied is limited at present by the relatively long time required to obtain and analyse the E.C.G. data. The use of a larger multichannel E.C.G. system would not only speed up the data acquisition but also improve the accuracy of the maps. Such an expansion would require on-line computing facilities capable of processing the larger amounts of data.

Such technical improvements may eventually lead to a system whereby the multiple E.C.G. signals can be obtained from the patient and the results displayed in a matter of minutes. This would allow more extensive studies from which it may be possible to build up diagnostic criteria similar to those now used in conventional electrocardiography. It seems likely that such multiple recordings from the thorax will form the basis of many future developments in electrocardiography.

REFERENCES

AMERICAN HEART ASSOCIATION (1967), 'Report of Committee on Electrocardiography', *Circulation*, **35,** 583.

HORAN, L. G., FLOWERS, N. C., and BRODY, D. A. (1963), 'Body Surface Potential Distribution: A Comparison of Naturally and Artificially Produced Signals as analysed by Digital Computer', *Circulation Res.*, **13,** 373.

NAHUM, L. H., MAURO, A., CHERNOFF, H. M., and SICKLAND, R. S. (1951), 'Instantaneous Equipotential Distribution on the Surface of the Human Body for Various Instants in the Cardiac Cycle', *J. appl. Physiol.*, **3,** 454.

SPACH, M. S., SILBERBERG, W. P., BOINEAU, J. P., BARR, R. C., LONG, E. C., GALLIE, T. M., GABOR, J. B., and WALLACE, A. G. (1966), 'Body Surface Isopotential Maps in Normal Children', *Am. Heart J.*, **72,** 640.

TACCARDI, B. (1963), 'Distribution of Heart Potentials on the Thoracic Surface of Normal Human Subjects', *Circulation Res.*, **12,** 341.

—— (1966), 'Body Surface Distribution of Equipotential Lines during Atrial Depolarization and Ventricular Repolarization', *Ibid.*, **14,** 865.

YOUNG, B. D. (1967), 'Isopotential Mapping of the Human Thorax', *Proc. of 5th DECUS European Symposium*, p. 133.

DISCUSSION

Question (Dr. G. A. Thompson): The heart is relatively simple in electrical terms. Is there any work done on electro-encephalograms and have you done any?

Answer: I am not aware of any applications of isopotential mapping to electro-encephalography. The main technical problem would be the relatively small size of the E.E.G. compared with the E.C.G. Also, the positioning of a sufficient number of electrodes on the head would be rather difficult.

May I also say that I do not regard the electrical processes of the heart as simple. They are complex, although less so than those of the brain.

Comment (J. H. Mitchell): Dr. Grey Walter has done a lot of work in this field.

Question (R. J. Sims): Is it possible for Mr. Young to give us any information on the effect the application of his technique has had on the management of patients?

Answer: This technique is still in the development stage and there is a great deal of research to be carried out before it can become a routine diagnostic procedure. However, I would say that, ultimately, the type of mapping techniques described in my lecture will become an important part of clinical electrocardiography.

Question (H. Norden): How does your technique compare with vector-cardiography?

Answer: I know of no directly comparative studies between vector-cardiography and isopotential mapping. Our view is that the two approaches will be complementary with vector-cardiography being used for routine reporting and isopotential mapping probably being applied to the more difficult cases.

Question (Professor J. Anderson): You referred in your lecture to anterior infarction. Have you also studied patients with posterior infarctions ?

Answer: The only results we have at the moment are for anterior infarctions although we are currently studying the effects of posterior infarctions.

Question (Professor J. G. Scadding): Have you applied your technique to cases other than infarctions, e.g. arrhythmias ?

Answer: We have only studied normal patients and those with infarcts, although I know that some workers are looking at other abnormalities of the heart. The application of this technique to arrhythmias would be extremely difficult since the data acquisition programme ideally requires a sinus rhythm.

Computer-assisted monitoring

J. M. Rawles

MONITORING has been defined as the acquisition, processing, display, and recording of physiological information from a hospital patient (Wolff, 1966). By this definition most monitoring is done by nurses, who measure a wide variety of physiological functions, some subtle and some not so subtle, some consciously, some almost subconsciously. Compared with the nurses' repertoire, the range of variables that can be monitored automatically by mechanical or electrical means is extremely limited. In the central nervous system there is the electroencephalogram and cerebrospinal fluid pressure. In the respiratory system, impedence spirometry gives the respiratory rate in anaesthetized patients and newborn babies. In other patients there are too many artefacts for it to be reliable. In the gastro-intestinal and urogenital systems, virtually nothing is monitored automatically, though a computer has been used to measure the urinary output in catheterized patients, which seems to me like taking a sledge hammer to crack a nut. Monitoring is, of course, used extensively in patients undergoing haemodialysis, but in this case it is the function of the machine, as much as the patient, that is monitored. It is in the cardiovascular system that automatic monitoring comes into its own with the measurement of intravascular pressures, the calculation of the cardiac output and peripheral resistance, and the recording, analysis, and display of the electrocardiogram.

I want to confine my observations now to the routine care of patients with myocardial infarction. It is in this all-too-common disease of the cardiovascular system that monitoring is having its greatest impact in general medical wards, and coronary care units up and down the country. Mortality figures are notoriously difficult to compare from unit to unit, but they are the best indication we have of the effectiveness of treatment. In those centres undertaking extensive monitoring of intravascular pressures, cardiac output, peripheral resistance, and in some cases computer analysis of results, it cannot be said that the mortality-rate is any lower than in those units where the bare minimum of monitoring is done, namely the display of the electrocardiogram (Aber, Portal, and Chopra, 1969). There is a definite difference, however, between coronary care units and general wards. What then is the essence of coronary care? It is the continuous observation of the patient and his electrocardiogram, backed up by staff who are immediately available and skilled in resuscitation and the treatment of arrhythmias. Such close surveillance is costly, and whereas a week's stay in a hospital bed on average costs £60, in a coronary care unit the cost is approximately twice this, the difference being due to the higher ratio of staff to patients (Oliver, 1971). It has been said (Wolff, 1968) that technology should be the great leveller, making good care available to the many, rather than performing miracles for the few, so with that in mind we must ask if the benefits of coronary care can be extended to those patients still admitted to general medical wards; and, we must ask if coronary care units can be run more economically using automatic and computerized monitoring equipment.

Let us look at some of the monitoring equipment in use today, and see how well it meets the need to draw attention to abnormalities of rate and rhythm in the electrocardiogram.

In *Fig.* 17 the electrocardiograph machine utilizes limb electrodes which are quite unsuitable for long-term monitoring. Limb electrodes are uncomfortable and placed so as to pick up the maximum amount of artefact due to muscular contraction. Chest electrodes, held in place by adhesive, are used now for long-term monitoring, but are still not ideal. The electrodes may become detached or the conducting jelly may dry out, so that poor contact is made and interference picked up. It should be emphasized that any sophisticated equipment for monitoring the E.C.G. is only as good as the connexion to the patient, the patient-machine interface.

Fig. 18 shows a patient attached by chest electrodes to an oscilloscope displaying the electrocardiogram. Most of us here are probably familiar with this equipment, Cardiac Recorders, 'Cardiorater', which the makers claim to have supplied to 70 per cent of the hospitals in the U.K. Most of us here are interested in sophisticated electronic equipment, and have some understanding of its workings. The average nurse, however, who will be using this, has little interest in electronic equipment, and less understanding. The most complex apparatus she will have met with is

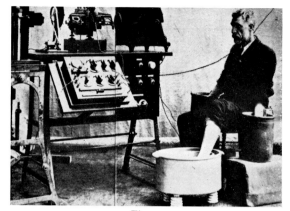

Fig. 17.

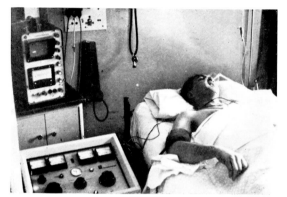

Fig. 18.

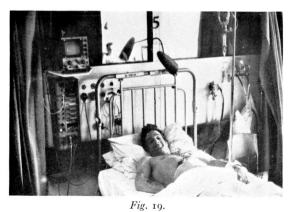

Fig. 19.

the television receiver, with only one-quarter of the number of
controls seen on this machine. For this equipment to work
properly under these circumstances, a thorough training scheme is
needed, and in practice is very difficult to organize. But that is by
the way. This equipment has an audible alarm, triggered by a
rate meter. Deviation of the recorded heart-rate outside pre-set
limits triggers the alarm with no delay. Unfortunately, movement
of the patient produces artefacts which are counted as QRS
complexes, and the heart-rate is apparently put up, producing a
false alarm. The electrodes, or the leads attached to the electrodes,
may become detached, also resulting in false alarms. We actually
counted the number of alarms that went off, and recorded how
many were true or false, and found that 91 per cent were false
(Rawles and Crockett, 1969a). Any nurse with experience of this
machine rapidly reaches a similar conclusion without so much
trouble, and turns the alarm off. In fairness to the makers, they
have now introduced a new version, which has fewer controls, and
an improved alarm system, though still operating on the same
principle. This slide also shows the Godart Haemotonograph,
which measures the blood-pressure automatically using an external
cuff. Even if there are no artefacts, and the pick up of the E.C.G.
is perfect, the value of such an alarm system is fairly limited.
If the limits on the heart-rate meter are set too close together,
physiological variation of the heart-rate will trigger the alarm
system and, if too far apart, important alterations of heart-rate will
not trigger the alarm, and neither will those serious dysrhythmias,
such as bursts of ventricular tachycardia, or frequent multifocal
ventricular extrasystoles, which are not associated with a gross
change of heart-rate. *Table I* shows the analysis of a series of
crises that occurred after myocardial infarction.

Table I.—CRISES FOLLOWING MYOCARDIAL INFARCTION

Dysrhythmias associated with gross change of heart-rate	35 per cent
Dysrhythmias not associated with gross change of heart-rate	35 per cent
Hypotension	10 per cent
Pain	10 per cent
Dyspnoea or apnoea	5 per cent
Other	5 per cent
Total	100 per cent

A crisis was defined as a deterioration in the patient's condition,
or the onset of a dysrhythmia that needed treatment to terminate

it: thus onset of multifocal ectopics, though not obviously associated with clinical deterioration, required treatment, and constituted a crisis. It can be seen that for every crisis from a dysrhythmia that would be expected to trigger a rate-operated alarm system, there was another, not associated with a gross change of heart-rate and not expected to trigger the alarm. Further, all crises due to dysrhythmias constitute only 70 per cent of the total, and there are other important causes of deterioration which are not initially reflected in any abnormality of the electrocardiogram.

If a patient with myocardial infarction and his E.C.G. is watched continuously by a nurse, then every crisis that occurs will be noticed and the doctor informed, that is an alarm raised, and every alarm will be the result of a crisis. The nurse then is a perfect monitor; every crisis resulting in an alarm and every alarm the result of a crisis, no false negatives or false positives. This is the ideal towards which the designers of automatic monitoring equipment are striving. The equipment just illustrated did not score well by these standards, only 35 per cent of crises triggering alarms, and only 9 per cent of the alarms being the result of the heart-rate deviating outside the pre-set limits, 91 per cent of the alarms being false. An even smaller proportion of the alarms, 3·5 per cent, actually resulted from a crisis, the other true alarms being the result of physiological variations in pulse-rate. In any alarm system, if the proportion of false alarms is too great, the alarm when it sounds evokes no sense of surprise or urgency, and goes unheeded. Further, if one patient is monitored, and there are six false alarms a day, this may be acceptable, but if there are six patients in the same area monitored, and there are 36 false alarms a day, this is unacceptable. Thus, the more patients there are monitored in an area, the better the alarm system has to be.

Fig. 19 shows a patient attached to the Monitron system of patient monitoring, which has been developed by the Medical Research Council Bio-medical Engineering Division. This has an E.C.G. display and an alarm system based on the heart-rate, and in addition an automatic blood-pressure machine with an external cuff, which was seen in *Fig.* 18. Fall of the systolic blood-pressure can also trigger an alarm. The complete system displays the current pulse-rate, blood-pressure and temperature at the nurses' station, and records these measurements on a chart. The circuitry of the heart-rate-operated alarm system is considerably more advanced than that in the Cardiorater, with an automatic gain control and efficient filter circuits to eliminate artefacts. Further, if the recorded heart-rate exceeds the pre-set limits, there is a 10-sec. delay before the alarm sounds. If the artefacts result from a patient turning over in bed, causing the recorded heart-rate to exceed the upper limit, the patient will have settled down again in the 10 sec. before the alarm is actuated. Many false alarms are thus avoided. Using the same criteria as with the Cardiorater, 65 per cent of the alarms were false, but, in fact, only 4·3 per cent of alarms resulted from a crisis. Forty-one per cent of crises triggered the alarm system (Rawles and Crockett, 1969b). This is an improvement on the cardiorater, but falls a long way short of perfection, for reasons outlined previously.

This is the background to the use of the computer in monitoring patients with myocardial infarction. How can the computer be expected to help ? An E.C.G. diagnostic service that is completely computerized is available in one American state, the electrocardiograms being transmitted by telephone. The programme took 100 man-years to write, but the computer is still sometimes fooled by the noises on the telephone lines (Caceres and Dreifus, 1970) and it is unable to diagnose the more complex dysrhythmias. In this system, the computer is only presented with clean E.C.G. information and not artefact-ridden electrocardiograms from restless, shocked patients. In such cases the recognition of the QRS complex may be difficult, let alone the recognition of P wave, whose amplitude is, even in a good recording, little above the noise level, and yet the recognition of the P wave is essential for complete diagnosis of dysrhythmias. Another problem results from the super-abundance of data which is produced by computer analysis. In some computer systems it is possible to have printouts of the amplitude and duration of each of the components of the E.C.G. cycle, together with calculated data such as heart-rate. Other systems classify QRS complexes by shape and size and plot histograms of their relative frequency. When this type of information is combined with data concerning intravascular pressures and cardiac output, and for good measure the temperature of the great toe, it is possible to be overwhelmed by the information altogether, and computerized monitoring is no longer a help, but a hindrance to good management (Osborn and others, 1968).

It is worth mentioning at this point a concept which originated in the field of business management. It is management by exception. In this type of business management, the highly-trained business executive sits at an empty desk, he plays no part in the routine running of the business, but should any trouble arise, it falls to him to sort it out. This, surely, should be the doctor's role in the coronary care unit. He should not be burdened with the wealth of normal data that is collected, but he should be notified of potentially serious deviations from normality.

It is important to recognize the differing requirements of computers for service needs and for research. In the former, the principal requirement is the recognition of life-threatening dysrhythmias. In the latter, there is a need for more detailed analysis and diagnosis of dysrhythmias, often in retrospect, using E.C.G. recordings stored on magnetic tape and replayed at high speed. Cost effectiveness is another consideration. Although there is clearly a role for the use of the computer to relieve nurses of the tedious task of continuously watching the E.C.G. on an oscilloscope, the possible saving in staff, however, is not that great, because there is still a need for a high staff-patient ratio for the institution of therapy and for general observation of the patient, apart from his electrocardiogram. Technically speaking, it would be fairly simple to devise means of giving treatment according to the results of computerized dysrhythmias diagnosis thus saving on staff, but with the present state of the art, D.C. shock therapy for example is better left at the discretion of nurses and doctors. A further consideration is whether it is better to have a large computer, time-shared, between a number of patients, or a small computer for each patient, though most of the work that has been done in this field has been done with the former system.

Now the most serious dysrhythmias are associated with profound bradycardia, marked tachycardia, or originate in the ventricles, namely, frequent multifocal ventricular ectopics, ventricular tachycardia, or ventricular fibrillation. This is fortunate for the designer of computerized monitoring equipment because it is relatively easy to detect changes in heart-rate or changes in the shape of the QRS complex that occur with ventricular dysrhythmias. I have recently, thanks to the generosity of the manufacturers, had some experience with a commercially-available device, the Hewlett-Packard Arrhythmia Monitor (*Fig.* 20). This is essentially a small, fixed programme hybrid computer. It is used in conjunction with a conventional bedside oscilloscope, and accepts a high level E.C.G. signal from one patient. No attempt is made to identify the P wave of the E.C.G.,

98

and the instrument concentrates on the QRS complex. A QRS complex is considered to be present if both the signal and its derivative exceed a certain threshold value at least 240 msec. after the previous QRS complex. The width of the QRS complex is determined from the derivative and is compared digitally with a reference width measurement stored during an initial 'store normal' sequence of a few seconds. During this sequence threshold values for the QRS complex and the derivative are also stored. There are a number of safeguards for the rejection of artefacts,

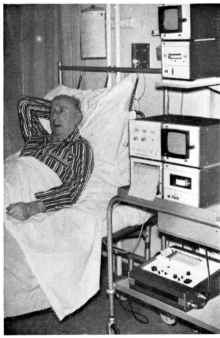

Fig. 20.

with filter circuits to reject low-frequency base-line wander, and also for rejection of high-frequency artefacts from muscle noise and supply line interference. Noise spikes narrower than 5–10 msec. are ignored by the logic and spikes not occurring close to the QRS complex are gated out. If there is an excessive number of excursions of the derivative, then an artefact is considered present, as it is when there is excessive base-line wander. When an artefact is deemed present, then categorization of the beats as normal, widened or premature, is inhibited. A widened QRS beat is one which exceeds the reference width by 15 msec., and a premature beat is one which occurs with an interval between its R wave and that of the preceding R wave, 20 per cent less than a recent running average of RR intervals. There are two alarm lights on the arrhythmia monitor, one is lit when a run of 3 or 6 ectopics is detected, widened beats triggering this alarm. The second alarm light is lit when the frequency of either widened or premature beats exceeds the pre-set limit of 6 or 12 per min. A third light comes on if an artefact is detected, and in this case there is inhibition of alarm circuits. An associated E.C.G. machine can be set to record either premature or widened beats, or both, or to record just when the alarms are lit. The E.C.G. record is taken from a 3-sec. tape loop, so recording events leading up to and including the alarm situation. An additional associated piece of equipment is the trend recorder, on which the heart-rate and ectopic frequency is recorded on slow-running paper at 1 cm. per hr.

On paper then, this instrument meets many of the requirements outlined above. It is small and portable. It is relatively cheap. In a patient with sinus rhythm, its only output is a short strip of paper from the trend recorder indicating the heart-rate and the frequency of ectopics. The alarms can be set to indicate life-threatening ventricular dysrhythmias, picked up because of widened beats. In patients who already have wide QRS complexes, because, for example, they have bundle-branch block, or are paced with an indwelling pacemaker catheter, extrasystoles can be detected because of the prematurity. In conjunction with a conventional rate-operated alarm system, the arrhythmias monitor should provide recognition of all important dysrhythmias, apart from, perhaps, second-degree heart-block not associated with bradycardia. The histogram of ectopic frequency on the trend recorder gives a very useful indication of the effectiveness of treatment to suppress ectopic activity, and can be correlated with the heart-rate.

Now, how does the equipment work in the clinical situation ? Its performance, in my hands, has been somewhat inconsistent. With some patients it behaved impeccably, doing just what was expected of it, but in other patients, for no apparent reason, time and time again an alarm would be indicated because runs of complexes were being categorized as widened. In a few patients, this defect could be cured by readjusting and resiting the chest electrodes, but some patients proved impossible to monitor reliably because of this shortcoming. The following illustrations show some examples of the arrhythmia monitor in action.

Fig. 21 shows part of the E.C.G. recorded automatically when the arrhythmia monitor picked up these supraventricular ectopics. The patient, in fact, had not had a coronary, but had been suffering from paroxysms of tachycardia of uncertain aetiology. It was suspected that these were, in fact, supraventricular in origin, and the alarms were set so that the E.C.G. machine would record frequent or runs of premature beats. Notice that the overall rate was not increased. Notice, also, that the ectopic beats, although slightly aberrant, are not widened, but are nonetheless picked up on account of their prematurity.

Fig. 22 shows the E.C.G. of the same patient a few moments later with a 4-sec. burst of atrial flutter, which was not noticed by the nursing staff on the monitor, nor by the patient. It would not have been noticed either by a conventional rate-operated alarm because it was of too short a duration, but its capture on this record enabled a diagnosis to be made with reasonable certainty.

Fig. 23 shows the onset of A–V junctional rhythm in a patient with a myocardial infarction. There is virtually no change of the heart-rate, as the patient changes from sinus rhythm to junctional rhythm, but the complexes are widened enough to trigger the arrhythmia monitor.

Fig. 24 shows some ventricular extrasystoles in a patient who, in addition, has atrial tachycardia with a variable block. These ectopics were detected because of their increased duration, but again there is no marked increase of heart-rate.

Fig. 25 shows a run of four multiform ventricular ectopics. In none of these examples, so far, would a conventional rate-operated alarm have detected any abnormality.

Fig. 26 shows the onset of ventricular tachycardia associated with an increased heart-rate from 100 to 130. This might have been picked up with a rate-operated alarm had it been set say at 120, pretty close to the normal rate, and very liable to be triggered by artefacts or by physiological variations of the heart-rate.

Fig. 27 shows part of the trend record of a patient with a myocardial infarction, the time scale running vertically on the right-hand side from below upwards. The patient was having rather frequent ventricular ectopics at 2 a.m. when a lignocaine infusion was commenced. During the night the frequency of the ectopics diminished. On the left is shown his heart-rate.

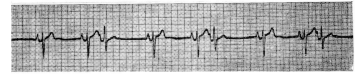

Fig. 21.

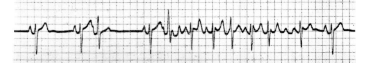

Fig. 22.

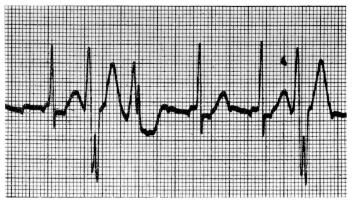

Fig. 23.

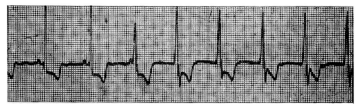

Fig. 24.

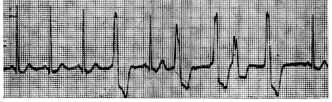

Fig. 25.

102

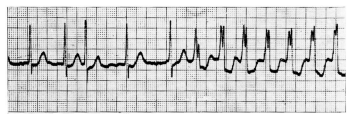

Fig. 26.

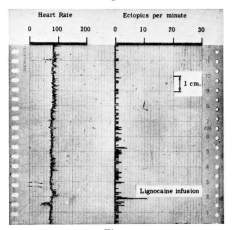

Fig. 27.

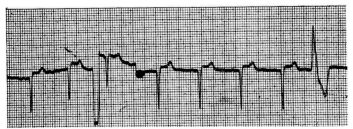

Fig. 28.

Now, we have seen what the Arrhythmia Monitor can do; let us look briefly at what it cannot do.

Fig. 28 shows on the left an artefact of dubious origin, which triggered the alarm on account of its breadth, and on the right of the record we see a ventricular ectopic. I think many of us would be hard put to say exactly why the wide bizarre deflection on the left-hand part of the record was not an ectopic, and would be daunted by the task of writing a computer programme to distinguish between the two.

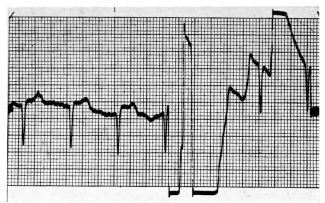

Fig. 29.

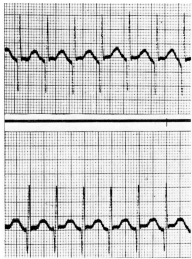

Fig. 30.

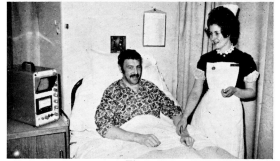

Fig. 31.

Fig. 29 shows a period of artefacts due to movement of the patient, which was not recognized as such by the artefact processor, and was classified as an arrhythmia.

The upper part of *Fig.* 30 shows the 'store normal' complexes from a patient, and below it complexes which were classified as widened, and triggered an alarm. Although minor differences between the two records can be distinguished, it is hard to say exactly why the record below was classed as abnormal. Excluding a few patients, such as the last, who proved impossible to monitor reliably for any period of time without getting false alarms triggered, the incidence of false alarms was 39 per cent of the total. It is not possible to say how many dysrhythmias were missed by the equipment, but judging by my experience of the arrhythmia monitor very few indeed would have failed to trigger one or other of the alarm systems.

In conclusion, this equipment is a worth-while advance in that it will detect automatically many dysrhythmias, which would not be detected by a conventional rate-operated alarm or even by nurses, unless they were exceptionally vigilant, and yet it is still associated with a high proportion of false alarms which limit its usefulness. Its possible role must also be seen in the perspective of the figures quoted earlier, namely that only 70 per cent of the crises that occur in patients with myocardial infarction are actually due to dysrhythmias. The other 30 per cent of crises would go undetected by the best E.C.G. monitor that could be devised.

In my opinion, then, even in 1971, the best monitor of them all is a nurse (*Fig.* 31), if you can get one.

REFERENCES

ABER, C. P., PORTAL, R. W., and CHOPRA, H. P. (1969), 'Cardiac Monitoring in a Regional Hospital', *Br. med. J.*, **1**, 209.

CACERES, C. A., and DREIFUS, L. S. (Eds.) (1970), *Clinical Electrocardiography and Computers*. London: Academic.

OLIVER, M. F. (1971), personal communication.

OSBORN, J. J., BEAUMONT, J. J., RAISON, J. C. and others (1968), 'Measurement and Monitoring of Acutely Ill Patients by Digital Computer', *Surgery, St. Louis*, **64**, 1057.

RAWLES, J. M., and CROCKETT, G. S. (1969a), 'Evaluation of Electrocardiogram Monitoring Apparatus on a General Medical Ward', *Biomed. Engin.*, **4**, 154.

— — — — (1969b), 'Automation on a General Medical Ward: Monitron System of Patient Monitoring', *Br. med. J.*, **3**, 707.

WOLFF, H. S. (1966), *J. Ass. Adv. med. Instrum.*, **1**, 50.

— — (1968), *Biomed. Engin.*, **3**, 17.

DISCUSSION

Question (Professor B. Lennox): It is disappointing that Dr. Rawles had to go to the U.S.A. for examples of distant analysis. We've had a computerized E.C.G. diagnostic service in Glasgow for some time.

Answer: Glasgow should get a better P.R.O.!

Question (Professor F. W. Donaldson): May not false alarms be eliminated by engineers, e.g., alarms due to patients turning over in bed?

Answer: There is in the Monitron system a 10-sec. delay, so that the number of false alarms has been greatly reduced. We are now working on the problem of detection of patients moving in bed, and inhibiting the alarms as long as movement continues.

Question (D. C. Manley): Have you considered the possibility of putting a patient on a cellular mattress to detect movement—we are working on this in Stoke-on-Trent.

Answer: My technique will be using a commercially available apnoea monitor which uses the same principle.

Some considerations in using the computer in the diagnostic X-ray department

H. Summers

BEFORE I begin the main substance of this talk, I must explain that I am not to be regarded as a radiologist. My viewpoint and position has been that of an administrator. It has been my task for some years to advise a Regional Hospital Board on the allocation and expenditure of money for X-ray departments, and I have contributed in material degree to forming opinion in that Board on the place of computers to be used for clinical, as distinct from administrative, purposes, and on what degree expenditure in that direction might be justified. Put shortly, my approach is 'What do we get for our money?' and 'Is it worth the cost?'

At the first conference held in Blackburn three years ago on 'Computers in Medicine', the theme was 'Where?', that is, where will the computer help? In the three intervening years we seem to have made good progress in answering that question: and the theme now seems to be 'How?' In X-ray matters, however, I think that we are still largely in the first phase; we are still asking 'Where?' I shall not attempt to give a comprehensive answer, but will instead discuss four fields of activity which might provide the answer to 'Where?' They are:—

1. Computer-assisted clinical diagnosis.
2. Computer-assisted administrative activities.
3. Computer-assisted radionuclide scanning.
4. Computer-assistance in radiation protection programmes.

1. THE PLACE OF THE COMPUTER IN RADIOLOGICAL DIAGNOSIS

There is something attractive about the idea that the computer could scan an X-ray film, and point out a diagnosis without human assistance. The film, after all, can be divided into a number of tiny imaginary squares, each of which could be examined in turn

107

for its degree of translucency or opacity, and the findings then added up and evaluated. Such a proposal invites a number of comments: the first is that the proposal implies that diagnosis is generally difficult and obscure. This is not so, and many diagnoses are obvious at a glance. Innumerable examples could be given, and the slides shown of various fractures, urinary tract calculi, and foreign bodies are merely a few examples. For such examples, a computer would be wasteful, and indeed something of a cumbersome burden. That the computer could calculate probabilities of the diagnosis being correct is also superfluous in many instances, where diagnosis is certain and unequivocal, and does not rest on probability.

The concept of diagnosis itself is worth a moment's consideration. Diagnosis is not a single indivisible item, the selection of a name. The abnormality in the patient is a process, and we need to know how far it has progressed and how rapidly, and whether there are any associated or distant consequences. Single phrases for an X-ray diagnosis like supracondylar fracture of the humerus, pyelonephritis, tuberculosis are quite insufficient as a basis for therapy.

There is thirdly the considerable variation of the normal, of which some examples are shown, and the further variation in appearance due to variations in film processing. All these can be allowed for almost instantaneously, by the trained eye and mind.

Let us not spend too much time on the possibility of computer scanning and reporting, and accept that its possibility does not seem likely to become reality in the foreseeable future. Would it then be practicable and desirable for the radiologist to look at the films, but instead of diagnosing, to describe the appearances, and to feed the information into the computer, which would then list diagnoses with their degree of probability. I am not talking here of such an application in specialized fields but, on the contrary, for the whole field of radiology. The idea, in my experience, is far more attractive to non-medical men than to those medical men who are actually concerned with practical diagnosis. The advantages of the computer are obvious: the accuracy of diagnosis is not limited by the knowledge and perspicacity of the particular radiologist, but the whole of accumulated information can be at his disposal. In addition, the past record of the particular patient under review can be stored in the machine, and compared, for investigative or statistical purposes, with records of other patients also fed into the computer.

To a practical radiologist to use such a system for *all* diagnosis seems unbelievably ponderous, time-wasting, and uselessly expensive. All the objections already made apply equally in this instance: the objections that the diagnosis is so often obvious; that it would take longer to fully describe the abnormality than to interpret and give a diagnosis; that the diagnosis might be certain and probabilities unnecessary; that a single name to a diagnosis is inadequate. Most relevant is the obvious point that the radiologist, if not sufficiently skilful, may fail to observe an abnormal finding. Of course, without the computer, the diagnosis will be equally at fault. The point, however, is that the computer requires accurate reporting. No computer can turn a poor radiologist into a good one, nor compensate for his deficiencies. The well-known phrase of 'garbage in, garbage out' is as true here as elsewhere. The objection could be met in material degree by using a long check list of items to be noted on the radiograph, but such a list is extraordinarily time-consuming if one has to make a verbal or written observation on each item instead of so quickly discarding the negative findings. Additionally much radiological material is non-numerical and somewhat subjective in character, and it would be a formidable task to digitize it and prepare it for the machine.

The next objection to be made is that the boundary between normal and abnormal is not always sharp, but may be diffuse. Lung appearances accepted as within normal limits in Manchester would be regarded as abnormal in Stockholm, and possibly in Aberdeen for that matter. In deciding in such instances what is to be put into the computer, the operator is already making his diagnosis, so why add the computer ? And in similar manner, not all disease entities are well defined, and there may be some overlapping, or one name may possibly cover several as yet unseparated conditions as we heard yesterday when ulcerative colitis was discussed.

Yet a further difficulty arises because some conditions are easily recognized at a glance, and yet are sufficiently rare that to include them in computer programmes would be an enormous labour. There is no problem in storing the information in the computer, but there is in the task and expense of writing the programme in the first place. Some examples are shown of such conditions as cysticercosis in the pectoral muscles, agenesis of a lung, carcinoma of the jejunum, and arteriovenous malformation of the forearm.

A final objection, and to my mind the most serious, and one which outweighs all the others put together, is the danger of fossilizing knowledge. Once the computer programme has been written, there will be reluctance to undertake the exceedingly laborious and most costly task of constantly modifying it to take in new knowledge, and knowledge whose accretion is not only in a few branches of medicine, but over the whole field. Furthermore, it is knowledge which does not consist only of new information to be added, but after a decade of such accumulation, to perhaps a complete revision of outlook, and the discarding of a sizeable proportion of that which has accumulated. The diagnosis of the several causes of bone cysts and the reinterpretation of metabolic bone diseases in terms of gastrointestinal or renal abnormalities are examples of the changing concepts; the great number of newly recognized inherited abnormalities is an example of accretion: the better understanding of immunology and the penetration of the information into the understanding of so many pathological processes illustrates both accretion and altered concepts. And, with reference to our main theme, once too much radiological skill has been lost, there is the possibility that problems needing investigation may not be so readily recognized: new work may not be undertaken because there is no awareness of the unsolved problem, and then the tendency towards fossilization of knowledge at its present state of development is still further emphasized.

Possibly my review so far may have been over-pessimistic, but in what I have said I have been speaking mainly to the non-medical computer expert, and not to the medical man, who would regard much of my account as self-evident. I have met so many non-medical computer men who are quite convinced that the computer is the answer to all the questions of diagnosis. I do want to convey to such experts that the matter of using computers generally for all types of diagnosis may not be possible: that if it is possible, there are formidable difficulties to be overcome before it is applied in practice: and that in any event, such use is far from being always necessary and advantageous, and may in the long run show very serious disadvantages. I would suggest to such workers that to follow this line may lead them along a sterile pathway, and that their energy and efforts would bring a better return if used to study other applications of the computer in medicine.

Having then discussed in some detail what I think the computer cannot do, I would like in the rest of this talk to examine topics where the computer has been, or shows great promise of being, of considerable assistance. In diagnosis itself the computer has in fact shown promise, but only when it has been applied in a limited field for the solution of certain specific problems, and it is perhaps in this type of application that it may prove of use. I am not hoping to be comprehensive, so will mention only two of a larger series of attempts, the two showing promise, and each being of rather a different nature. The first use is to estimate the intensity of bone mineralization: such changes are detectable visually only when the calcium content has changed by at least 25–30 per cent. Considerably smaller changes in bone density can be detected quite accurately, however, by passing the film through an optical scanning system which measures light transmission, and then analysing the readings with a small digital computer. The exposure of the film and the processing must be carefully standardized. As said earlier, this is hardly feasible on a large scale, but with considerable care by the operator, it can be done on a small scale, and the method has been used with success by Vogt and his colleagues in Texas.

The second example will be considered in more detail because it illustrates well what is involved both in writing a computer programme, and in reading an X-ray film with a view to using that programme. Where a brain tumour is suspected, the radiologist will look for clear evidence of its presence, and if he cannot obtain this by one method of investigation, e.g., angiography, he will try another method, e.g., pneumography. Nevertheless the angiographic films may provide a considerable amount of information, despite their falling short of giving all that is desired: it is possible that a more exhaustive examination may in fact give the diagnosis, and then there would be no need to have recourse to the subsequent examination of pneumography. Du Boulay (du Boulay and Price, 1968), of St. Bartholomew's Hospital, London, analysed the angiographic findings of perisellar tumours, and observed that although the major signs of tumour may be lacking, certain combinations of minor signs were strongly suggestive of the diagnosis. It is, however, difficult to work out theoretically in advance what these combinations were, and perhaps even more difficult for the radiologist, once the combinations were known, to retain them in his memory for long periods of time. Comprehensive check lists of changes were made therefore, each change being a single definable sign, such as erosion of a particular bone feature, expansion of the deep part of the internal auditory meatus, soft-tissue swelling in the nasopharynx, and so on; each such defined sign was called a test. The significance of the tests, singly and in various combinations, was worked out by the computer by cross checking with the precise diagnosis when the latter became available, at operation or autopsy. Du Boulay drew up 8 tables of Comprehensive Tests, one table for each of the 8 techniques that might be used for diagnosing perisellar tumours. Omitting technique 8 on scanning, there were between 18 and 88 basic tests in each table, and about 400 tests in all. A disease index was also prepared; it was found difficult to decide upon a suitable classification, as even a full histological examination did not invariably give a certain and conclusive answer as to which was the predominant tumour cell: however, 186 possible varieties were eventually listed in the classification, taking into account anatomical site, pathological type, and prognostic future. All this information, about 140,000 items in all, was placed on one reel of magnetic tape, which could be scanned by the computer in less than one minute. Diagnoses were given with their probabilities. To prevent the probabilities from being too close together, it was necessary to give a weighting to positive as opposed to negative signs, and to certain signs which were direct rather than secondary evidence of tumour, and yet again to some signs which appeared frequently and were associated with a particular lesion. Preliminary results only have been reported so far: a full report is promised when 1000 cases have been recorded. In the preliminary report, the first choice diagnoses have almost always correctly predicted the anatomical site, and have been correct on the pathological aspects in about half the cases, the second and third choices being correct pathologically in about another 20 per cent. Most of the errors are related to the paucity of material, an unusual case swaying the prediction to an unjustifiable degree: accumulation of information from more patients may therefore reduce these errors. Du Boulay concludes that the computer in no way can replace the observer, for each sign in the check list must be thought about and accurately assessed. In this limited series, in at least one case, the computer gave a better diagnosis than did the radiologist.

2. THE PLACE OF THE COMPUTER IN THE ADMINISTRATION OF THE X-RAY DEPARTMENT

To my knowledge, the computer has not been used in the administration of the X-ray department, at least in this country, nor abroad for other than recording financial charges. Possibly this is a consequence of conservatism, and because no great dissatisfaction has been expressed, X-ray departments apparently being run reasonably effectively. There are four factors: the patient, the films, the staff, and the paper records, and these must come together in various combinations at the appropriate times. An average district hospital may carry out of the order of 100,000 examinations in a year, most examinations taking more than one film. There is thus scope for computer assistance with the storage and recording of this considerable amount of information. The problems resemble those of pathology departments, about which a great deal has been written. I have no new thoughts to offer on X-ray department administration and will not spend time reviewing what has been established in pathology departments. But it can be said that the accumulated knowledge and experience are such as to assure successful function of any computerized administration introduced into an X-ray department. Industrial experience of stores management could also be applied to X-ray materials, of which there is an unexpectedly wide variety, so that stores could be maintained at minimal level, yet obviating any risk of going short.

3. COMPUTERS AND RADIO-ISOTOPE SCANNING

I turn now to the third of my major topics, the use of computers in radio-isotope scanning procedures. The application of isotopes in medical practice depends on the principle, true for all practical purposes, that a substance in which an isotope is incorporated is treated by the body as if it were the normal substance. Where the isotope is radioactive, radiation will be emitted, and can be recorded by suitable means. In a normal organ, the radio-isotope will take up a particular distribution; in an abnormal organ, a variant of this, which variant may have diagnostic value. Suitable radio-isotopes and appropriate techniques are now available for the examination of most organs of the body. Suitable recording devices will, of course, be needed to detect and estimate the radiation given off. X-ray film can be used here, as elsewhere, but is insensitive and would have to be placed in situ for unacceptably long periods. The emitted gamma-rays are therefore picked up by a suitable scintillation crystal, in which the ray produces an ionization, which in turn leads to an amplified pulse, to be either counted or recorded as a dot on a screen or card. The ideal would be to cover simultaneously the whole area under examination, and this is possible by simultaneously picking up from a number of suitably sited scintillation crystals, connected in turn to a recording camera. Despite much development work, however, I think it fair to say that at present no camera combines both good sensitivity and good resolution. The preferable technique therefore is by scanning: a single crystal reviews a small portion of the area under examination, and is moved to and fro over the whole area, recording from each portion in turn, and gradually building up the picture. Marks are made on the recording paper when gamma radiation enters the crystal. Usually an array of dots is printed, few dots where radiation is scanty, many dots where it is intense: some prefer to use different coloured dots to indicate different concentrations.

Now radioactive decay is a random process, and not one which is spread out perfectly evenly over a period of time. Thus errors of statistical uncertainty arise, and although the activity of the material may be fixed, the measured counts of this activity will vary between different but equal time periods. Where a count is made only once, it is generally too high or too low. Naturally the fluctuation is small where a large number of counts is made, and equally the statistical uncertainty becomes smaller as the size of the count increases. There are, however, obvious disadvantages to increasing the size of the count in an effort to improve accuracy: if a large dose of radio-isotope is given, the dose of radioactivity received by the patient begins to approach the undesirable level: and if the count is prolonged in time, the patient suffers discomfort. Thought has therefore been given as to how the computer can improve accuracy.

As I am not trying to be comprehensive, I shall describe only one of the attempted solutions, although in fact, the matter is under examination in other centres also. Popham and his colleagues in London began with the premise that conventional methods of recording scans may not always, because of statistical fluctuations, show a recognizable difference between the abnormal region and its more normal surroundings. Numerical analysis of data might therefore detect abnormalities which would otherwise be missed. This group of workers, when examining brain scans, therefore compared the area under examination with a known normal area, using statistical testing and computer analysis. There were a number of difficulties to overcome, and the application of computerized statistical analysis was not quite straightforward. Finding a normal standard was one: the unaffected side of the brain was used for anteroposterior scans. But for lateral scans, there was no really satisfactory normal base, and the affected region was compared with the more nearly normal areas of the same scan, or to my mind a less satisfactory method, was compared with an average count and pattern taken from a series of normal scans. Even so, there remained about 20 per cent of their patients who could not be evaluated by this technique, whether because of unsatisfactory alinement of the head, or because the head was of unusual shape; however, suggestions for overcoming these last problems have been made. These points are mentioned to show that attempted use of the computer is not always a simple process, but may introduce problems of its own. Popham and others (1970) comment that it is not possible to compare purely computer results with purely visual results, because clinical information about the patient is necessarily given to the examiners. Even so, considerable assistance was given by the computer in about 10 per cent of the patients examined. It would appear that the place of the computer will be to help, not with all diagnoses, but with that minority which are equivocal.

Another and quite different way of using the computer, which is not concerned primarily with the statistical variations, is to build up three-dimensional scans. The scanner is used in a type of tomograph action in which all the dots are out of focus, except those of one particular horizontal layer of the body. Scans are taken with different horizontal layers in focus, and the separate scans in focus are summed up by computer to give a three-dimensional picture, and to provide understanding of what is happening in any particular small volume of the whole.

4. RADIATION PROTECTION AND THE COMPUTER

I now come to radiation protection, my final topic where the computer would find an application, and indeed where what I shall propose would perhaps not be possible otherwise.

X-rays have great penetrative power, causing injury deep in the body as well as on the surface. Given in large doses over a short period, X-rays lead to skin burns and radiation sickness, and in those who survive, to a subsequent increased incidence of tumours. However we are not concerned here with massive short-term exposure, but the effects of successive small doses, whose administration is spread out over a long period of time, as when a person receives a diagnostic X-ray examination from time to time. Two questions follow: what disadvantageous sequelae, if any, may follow from such radiation ? and how much radiation is acceptable before the risk becomes significant ? Taking the first question, the injurious effects of long-term intermittent low-radiation dosage are not seen until months or years later, and there is a latent period during which all appears well. The major consequences may be classified as follows:—

1. *To the Foetus:*—
    a. 50 rads in the early weeks lead to congenital defects.
    b. 1000 rads may lead to abortion.
    c. There is an increased incidence of childhood malignancy.

2. *To the Body of the Individual:*—
    a. 400 rads leads to destruction of haemopoietic tissue.
    b. 200 rads may lead to leukaemia.
    c. There are changes in the eyes (cataracts) and in the skin, lungs, and bones.

3. *To the Gonads and Germ Cells:*—
    a. *Beneficial mutations* are too rare to need consideration.
    b. *Debilitating mutations* may be compatible with survival to reproductive age, when the defective genetic heritage will be transmitted to yet another generation. Once in the chromosome, on the accepted view, the damage will remain for many generations, perhaps hundreds of years, possibly for ever. This type of damage is the social danger.
    c. *Very serious chromosome damage.* The progeny possesses defects incompatible with life. This is a disaster to the individual, and to his parents, but not to his descendants, as there are none.
    d. *Permanent sterility.* May be caused by doses of 500 rads.

The social danger to future generations, and the harmful effects to society are predominantly in consequence of the introduction of debilitating mutations.

Our second question was to ask how much radiation is acceptable ? How much radiation, averaged out over the whole community, will produce harmful mutations with sufficient frequency to be a social hazard ? Before answering this, we should remind ourselves that it is not possible to entirely escape radiation, for small doses reach us from natural sources, and by the age of 30 years, that is, by the end of the main reproductive period, have amounted in total to 3–4 rads, as shown in *Table II*.

To return to the question, clearly any assessment of social hazard is arbitrary, and some would say that *any* additional debilitating mutations, no matter how few, are undesirable. The Adrian Committee's final report of 1966, and the authoritative I.C.R.P. (International Committee for Radiation Protection) Publication No. 16, of 1969, are both prepared to draw the line at a doubling of the natural mutation rate, and to say that any frequency of harmful mutation higher than this, is unacceptable.

Table II.—TYPICAL DOSAGE FROM NATURAL SOURCES: CONCEPTION TO 30 YEARS OF AGE

SOURCE OF RADIATION	DOSE IN RADS	
	To the Gonads	*To Bone-marrow*
Cosmic rays	1·50	1·50
Terrestial radiation	1·50	1·50
Internal radiation ^{40}K, ^{14}C, ^{226}Ra, ^{228}Ra, ^{222}Ra	0·75	0·69
Totals	3·75	3·69

The amount of radiation required to produce such a doubling has been variously estimated at an average of 10–100 rads per person spread over the first 30 years of life. This is an average figure of the total radiation from all sources, natural, diagnostic, industrial, divided by the figure for the size of the population. Nobody knows beyond doubt whether there is any recovery between intermittent doses, but no one claims that it is more than partial, if it does take place. This is a most significant conclusion, for it implies that the effects of radiation are inevitably cumulative. The doses add up year by year, and the only effect of recovery, if it occurs, is to delay the accumulation.

Opinions also differ as to whether there is a threshold which has to be reached before damage occurs, but if one exists it is undoubtedly a low one. The same I.C.R.P. Publication No. 16 states that 'there may be no lower limit for the initiation of deleterious effects. A cell affected by small doses of radiation may develop malignant neoplasia or chromosomal aberration.'

It may be concluded then without serious error that probably all radiation is deleterious, that there is possibly no lower limit below which there is safety, and that the dosage is cumulative. Against this we offset the undoubted benefits of properly conducted diagnostic examinations, but ask whether there is an upper limit to the total amount of diagnostic radiation permissible by the age of 30 ? Again it must be said that we are concerned with the average amount per member of population, that is with the total dosage of all diagnostic radiation divided by the total population. We are examining the social problem, not the individual one. More than

Table III.—Dose Received During X-ray Examinations

EXAMINATION	Dose in Millirads		
	Gonad Dose		Mean Bone-marrow Dose Either Sex
	Males	Females	
Low Dose			
Head, limbs, chest	10	10	10–200
Moderate Dose			
Barium meal	50	150	300
High Dose			
Pelvis: hip	1000	350	50–200
Barium enema	200	800	600
Excretory urogram	1200	700	800
Urethrocystogram	200	1500	300

Table IV.—Frequency of X-ray Examinations

COUNTRY	YEAR	ANNUALLY PER 1000 OF POPULATION			
		Medical	M.M.R.	Dental	Total
U.K.	1957	280	95	40	415
Japan	1960–4	449	445	14	908
U.S.A.	1964	530	87	288	925
Switzerland	1957	640	190	140	970
Sweden	1966	470	105	580	1155

ever in this field of incomplete knowledge, any decision must be arbitrary. We have mentioned already that a dose in the range 10–100 rads is considered to be the mutation doubling dose. The Adrian Committee was prepared to accept a figure of twice the natural radiation, i.e., a total of 6 rads, as the maximum dose, additional to natural radiation, and averaged over the population, to be received by the age of 30. This is a quite arbitrary figure, but the Committee was a most able one, and it is preferable to work to a reasonable and thought out arbitrary figure than to none at all. The I.C.R.P. was in fact more cautious, and gave an upper limited of 5 rads.

The next and crucial question is to ask how near we are to reaching this figure. We need information on the amount of radiation received during an X-ray examination, and on the frequency of examinations. This information is given in the *Tables III* and *IV*.

The figures do show quite clearly that in advanced countries, in the late 1950s and early 1960s, each person was receiving of the order, on the average, of one X-ray examination each year.

The Adrian Committee estimated that by 1960, the mean annual gonad dose in the U.K., received from diagnostic radiation, was 0·032 mrads per person, or about 1 rad in 30 years. X-ray usage is increasing constantly, and it can be only a matter of time before U.K. usage has reached the Swiss level, if it has not already done so, which would indicate a total average dosage by the age of 30 of 2 or even more rads. This is a modest estimate, not an exaggerated one, and made with our feet firmly on the ground. It is, however, of the same order as the 5 rads maximum proposed by the I.C.R.P., and the 6 rads of the Adrian Committee.

The Adrian Committee in their original report of 1957 had suggested that changes in radiographic technique could in fact reduce the mean dose to about 20 per cent of what it was. No full-scale official survey has been made to see if their recommendations had been put into practice, but a limited private survey by Matthews and Miller in the Sheffield region in 1964 showed an increase in radiographic procedure per head of population of 26 per cent over the previous seven years, but nevertheless a fall in mean annual genetic dose because of improved techniques, such as the use of better beam filtration, gonad shields and light beam diaphragms. Nevertheless, over the three years 1957 to 1960, the Adrian Committee found, on the contrary, that mean annual dose had increased.

From these reports, we may conclude:—

    a. There is doubt about what the mean annual dose really is.
    b. There are grounds for believing, however, that although it is less than the 5 or 6 rads total in 30 years variously given

by authoritative bodies, the dosage may be a figure approaching the same order.

c. The long-term consequences of excessive radiation, disturbing generations to come, are so serious that, as a first stage, more accurate records of dosage received are essential. A watch can then be kept on what is happening, but the information must be obtained well in advance, for we dare not be overtaken by events.

It is here that the computer can make possible a scheme that otherwise might not be practicable. It would appear essential to have long-term records of the X-ray examinations of a sizeable population, and perhaps desirable to have such records for everybody in the country. My suggestion is to take a selected region of 2 or 3 million people, and to keep records of all the X-ray examinations which they receive. Without a computer this would be impossibly laborious, but with a computer no problem. People have no great difficulty in supplying their N.H.S. number to make an insurance claim, and equally they would not be X-rayed, save in emergency, without this number: they could in fact be told to bring their medical card when coming for an X-ray examination.

Ideally the dose received by the patient should be measured during each examination, and then added to his accumulated dose to date kept in the computer records. There is unfortunately no quick and simple means of measuring radiation dose accurately. There is equipment to do it, and it is precise and readily available, but its use is tricky, and needs a physicist. Initially therefore, and until simpler means of measurement are developed, it would be necessary to use average figures for the particular examination. This is clearly less accurate than a system of measurement made during the examination, but nevertheless would give information incomparably in advance of that which we have at present. It would of course be a simple task for the computer to calculate any mean annual dose rates, or other figures desired.

Should this system of keeping records of accumulated X-ray dosage prove feasible in a limited population, there would appear to be grounds for extending the scheme to the whole country. At present we are working, if not quite in the dark, certainly in the gloom. We have some vague idea of the average amount of gonad radiation received per head of the population, but no really accurate figures. We do not know what is the upper limit. Yet the consequences of error are so serious, and so irremediable.

Thought should be given to the desirability of keeping comprehensive records: the computer would appear to be an essential instrument if they are to be kept.

CONCLUSIONS

In this talk, I have reviewed some of the possible uses of the computer in the diagnostic radiology department as the matter presents itself to the administrator concerned with recommending the purchase if justified. I have not attempted to be comprehensive, and there are other uses for the computer which I have not reviewed, notably perhaps the recording and storage of diagnoses. I have tried to put out a few ideas about where I think the computer could be applied with benefit, and to mention others where I think that the pathway is sterile. For diagnosis, the computer might help in a limited number of restricted fields where difficult problems are common, but I do not think that the evidence so far amounts to more than a belief that further study is worth while: we are far from the stage where computers should be provided on a wide scale to deal with these problems. On a wider scale, I consider that to attempt to replace the radiologist by a computer is not only impossible, but also undesirable, and for the suggestion to be advocated is an implied admission by the supporter that he does not really understand how a diagnosis is made. For administrative work, I would wholeheartedly support the use of the computer. In connexion with scanning, again I would conclude that more evidence should be accumulated, but that the case for a computer appears materially stronger than for its use in difficult diagnostic problems. Lastly for radiation protection, the computer is an essential, if you think, as I do, that the time has come to begin the maintenance of individual radiation exposure records.

A paper such as this cannot be prepared without assistance, and I would like to acknowledge the help given to me by Mr. K. Bray, Dr. J. B. Fawcitt, and Miss J. Perry of Crumpsall Hospital, Manchester, and by Drs. Ian Isherwood and R. G. Ollerenshaw of Manchester Royal Infirmary. The opinions expressed are, of course, my own.

REFERENCES

Du Boulay, G., and Price, V. E. (1968), 'The Diagnosis of Intracranial Tumours assisted by Computer', *Br. J. Radiol.*, **41,** 762.
Popham, Mary G., Bull, J. W. D., and Emery, E. W. (1970), 'Interpretation of Brain Scans by Computer Analysis', *Ibid.*, **43,** 835.

DISCUSSION

Question (S. Sweenie): One cannot discount people over 30 years of age. Thus 17 per cent of births in Glasgow are to women over 35 years of age, and 30 per cent are to women over 30.

    Answer: The proposal that the age of 30 be regarded as the upper age for the main reproductive period is widely accepted, but if there is a sizeable population reproducing over this age, the dangers of debilitating mutations, as a consequence of total absorbed radiation to date, become that much more serious.

Question (Dr. D. M. Goldberg): While visiting the French centre for the analysis of ionizing radiation, I found that they had discovered a strict relationship between chromosome changes and exposures in the range of 10–100 rads.

    Answer: This is perfectly credible and acceptable, and again strengthens the case which I have put forward that the danger now may be greater than we think, and the need to begin to keep records more pressing.

Question (Dr. D. M. Goldberg): Why not have this in the U.K.? Pressure ought to be put on authorities to achieve this.

    Answer: I would very much like to see it.

Question (Dr. D. J. Roberts): Do you know of any beneficial mutations induced by X-rays?

    Answer: I don't know of any in man.

Question (Professor J. Anderson): What about the new varieties of wheat and rice?

    Answer: I am not familiar with these myself.

Comment (Dr. J. Rose): While the short-term advantages of the new varieties of cereals may be considerable, in the long run the replacement of hundreds of varieties by one or two may prove disastrous in the event of a disease attacking the plants.

Question (Professor F. W. Donaldson): Perhaps radiologists could set limits for film densities and thus be able to diagnose better by using improved parameters.

    Answer: This could be, but the computer will not help here, because of the practical impossibility of adequately standardizing exposure and development techniques.

Question (G. Pilling): There is a move to produce more accurate records of radiation given by using semi-automatic densitometers. This would produce better protection for radiologists.

    Answer: This is an encouraging development. The computer, in fact, is more use for protection, via sound records, than for diagnosis.

Computer applications in clinical biochemistry

A. Fleck, D. Reekie, and R. B. Marshall

IN recent years many descriptions and reviews of computer applications in clinical biochemistry laboratories have appeared (Griffiths and Carter, 1969; Whitehead, 1969; Abernethy and others, 1970; Hicks, Gieschen, Slack, and Larson, 1966; Hjelm, 1969). In this paper an attempt will be made to assess the benefits of different approaches, incidentally providing the rationale for our system. Since the work of most large clinical biochemistry laboratories is basically similar a brief description of the work flow through a laboratory provides the basis for discussion of the application of data processing or computer techniques at each stage.

In common with the other branches of laboratory medicine the work of the biochemistry laboratory results from the interaction of patient and doctor which leads in this case to a specimen and a request form. These items then pass through some form of transport system to the laboratory. The first stage of the work in the laboratory includes inspection to ensure matching and adequacy of sample and request form, then follows the analytical process which will be referred to as Stage 2, the checking of the report as Stage 3, and the final preparation of the report and despatch to the clinician as Stage 4.

Obviously patient and specimen identification are vital parts of this process. In order to return an adequate report fairly full particulars of the patient are required, for example, surname and forename or initials, date of birth, sex, hospital number and ward. Within the laboratory it is common practice to add an accession number both to the form and to the specimen. This permits adequate identification on worksheets and so on using the surname and the accession number alone, and has the combined advantages of reducing both the possibility of transcription errors and the amount of material to be written or read.

123

Such 'data condensation' facilitates the preparation of work sheets, an essential preliminary to Stage 2, the analysis.

Scale, or the amount of work done, is relevant at this point. A few larger laboratories such as ours process about half a million results a year from about 100,000 specimens.

The average number of specimens per day is about 400, comprised of 250 electrolytes, (i.e., plasma sodium, potassium, chloride, bicarbonate, and urea), 100 liver-function tests (bilirubin, alkaline phosphatase, and the transaminases, glutamate amino transferase and alanine amino transferase), and 50 miscellaneous (including serum calcium, phosphorus, proteins, etc.). These rough figures are subject to considerable fluctuation. For example, on Saturday mornings only about 100–200 specimens are received; during February–March and November the average work done in some days is about twice that in some days in July. In addition, there has been for many years a considerable annual growth of 20–25 per cent in the West of Scotland which shows no sign of slacking off due to the introduction of new techniques. It follows that planned capacity for work must allow a factor of about 6 times increase in 5 years. An additional factor pertinent to laboratory data processing is that specimens and request forms may arrive at the laboratory in batches of up to 90 or more at a time. Thus in a laboratory in which the data must be converted to a machine readable form at Stage 1, delays may occur due to the necessary data preparation steps (punching cards or tape and producing work sheets). This data-preparation step is at present one of the major problem areas in most laboratory data processing units because of the general lack of coherent hospital records and data processing systems. Cards pre-punched with the patient's identification data are in use in some hospitals. However, these and 'port-a-punch' cards are not entirely successful because a number are damaged before arrival in the laboratory and the data has to be re-punched (Baird and Garfunkel, 1965). Also to obtain a working system, patient admission must be organized so that data is prepared before the patient is transferred to the ward, and appropriate numbers of machine-readable request cards are sent to the ward preferably with the patient. Possibly the best system which can be envisaged at present requires a time-sharing laboratory computer linked to a hospital data bank and visual display units. With this equipment the doctor needs only to indicate the tests by marks on a computer-prepared laboratory requisition form from which on arrival at the laboratory the receptionist keys in the patient's identification number and checks that the visual display of full patient data is correct, after which the tests requested are keyed in using simple codes. Such a system is being developed in Boston (U.S.A.) (Katona, Pappalardo, Marble, Barnett, and Pashby, 1969).

In our own system patient data are entered by paper tape punched on Creed Envoy 'Electronic Dataprinters' in the laboratory. Once the data have been read into a computer with a suitable backing store several useful lists can be obtained very rapidly. These include centrifuging and sample allocation lists, work sheets, and lists of work not completed. The work sheet forms the link between Stage 1 and Stage 2, the analytical process. Any delays in preparing the work sheet lead to delays in setting up analytical systems, so that suitable backing stores such as disks or addressable magnetic tape are necessary; large conventional tape decks are less suitable than disks because of the non-sequential nature of the data presentation.

Much of the second stage of the process, the analytical work, is mechanized. In this country this amounts to about 80 per cent in the larger laboratories and although there are a variety of mechanized systems of analysis the bulk of the work is carried out using Technicon AutoAnalysers. With this equipment 40 samples (including standards, controls, and patient's specimens) are loaded in cups on a special tray, presented to a sampler which samples at a rate of 60 per hour, and the results appear as peaks on a potentiometric strip chart recorder. The data processing problems presented at this stage are, first, sample identification and, secondly, data acquisition.

The identification of samples (standards, controls, and patients' specimens) is commonly achieved by sequence or cup number which corresponds with that of the worksheet (Griffiths and Carter, 1969). Some systems permit corrections and substitution of specimens. This method is cheap and easily manipulated by technicians although liable to error. Positive sample identification which also presents few problems to technicians is in contrast expensive and is not liable to error. An early system of positive sample identification employed stub cards on which were printed a 5-digit number; these small cards were attached to the specimen tube which was then loaded on to a special Technicon sampler with a mechanical card-reading device attached (Rappoport,

Gennaro, and Constandse, 1968). More recently an optical character reading device has been displayed which achieves the same purpose of linking the specimen result to the specimen number within the mechanized analytical system.

Data acquisition is the area in which the greatest variety of work has been done. Methods of data acquisition vary from the simple manual procedures to potentiometric or curve-fitting trace readers, to analogue devices, which may include peak-picking and function generators and give a print-out of concentration, and finally to on-line computer systems.

In some circumstances it may be necessary to prepare manually read results in tape or punch card form for computer processing. Because this tends to be time consuming a good reason must exist for this procedure. The simplest and cheapest method of obtaining results from chart recorders in machine-readable form is to use a chart or trace reader. Several of these are available; among the simplest is that manufactured by the Chemical Electronics Co. of Durham (Dawson, Milner, and Mawston, 1969). It is a simple Y plotter and can by means of easily calibrated function generators give directly a printed list of concentration against sequence number or punch results on paper tape. Several other trace readers are available, for example those manufactured by Normalair Garrett and by D-mac. At present we use the Min-Mac, a less sophisticated (and cheaper) version of the D-mac trace reader. Although this equipment does not contain a function generator the output format can be changed by means of a plug board, additional identifying digits and characters can be added by means of a keyboard, and it can be linked directly to instruments such as computers, programmable calculators, or paper tape punches. We have used the Min-Mac coupled directly to the Wang 370 calculator to give direct read out of results from AutoAnalyser tracings (Tilstone and Fleck, 1970). This is very accurate and rapid, particularly when peak values only are read in. Alternatively, the values can be punched onto paper tape and the final results calculated directly by computer. This off-line computer approach is simple, cheap, reliable, and fast, and does not disrupt the normal work of the laboratory during its introduction. We have checked on the precision of the Min-Mac and in general use a standard deviation of 0·12 per cent T was obtained which is very satisfactory.

Some laboratories at present utilize 'On-line' data acquisition computer systems. These vary from systems which achieve not a great deal more than data acquisition and print out of a valid result to systems in which on-line patient data input is attempted in addition to on-line data acquisition and final reporting. Manufacturers of equipment at present in use in 'on-line mode' in Clinical Biochemistry Laboratories in this country include Elliot (903), Digital (PDP12), although the PDP8 and Linc 8 have also been used, and IBM (1130). Doubtless many other small computers would be applicable, including some of the Honeywell and Varian range and developments with Computer Technology's Modular one are awaited with interest.

Linking the computer to the AutoAnalyser requires some hardware. Two approaches are available, the first makes use of a retransmitting slidewire and with the second which requires buffer amplifiers, etc., the link is made directly to the colorimeter. In each, some form of channel identification and usually voltage calibration, etc., is required. Analogue to digital conversion is also necessary and usually high-quality cables to prevent electrical interference. After initial setting up, the equipment used in this area seems to give little trouble.

Perhaps surprisingly, the calculation of the initial results has been tackled in a variety of ways. Theoretically quantitative colorimetric methods should yield an exponential relationship between colour and concentration (Beer's law—concentration equals constant times (2-log per cent T) where per cent T refers to per cent transmission of light through the solution). However, for a variety of reasons this relation does not hold for all methods currently in use, although in our experience it does apply over a slightly restricted concentration range for the majority of methods. The restriction of the concentration range may not be so disadvantageous as might seem initially because at the limits of the per cent T scale the possible error becomes unacceptably large. Our investigations show that the use of the Beer's law relationship simplifies the calculation of the final result and leads to greater reliability because least squares methods can be applied readily to standard curves. We have also examined polynomial fitting to standard curves and find that there is little to be gained by going beyond the second order.

An alternative, used in the Elliot 903 systems, is linear interpolation. This follows, almost exactly, the manual chart reading approach, and seems to work well in practice. However, it seems to us unfortunate not to attempt to use the calculating power of

127

the computer to obtain a statistical (least squares) fit to a function which in addition to giving the fastest calculation of the sample result can also give some indication of its reliability. For completeness some mention must be made of recent developments by IBM. It seems that they are offering as an alternative to their rather expensive off-line data acquisition system (the 1080 used for example in Uppsala) the recently announced 'system 7' which is to be a small on-line computer system which could be linked to an 1130.

An advantage of on-line systems is that they can check whether a peak is valid or not before processing it further; that is, it must occur within the appropriate time limits and be of appropriate shape before it is accepted (Whitby and Simpson, 1969). This is a form of 'quality control' which is done with only poor sensitivity and high risk of error when done manually.

Table V.—SCOTTISH WRHB BIOCHEMISTRY LABORATORY COMPUTER SYSTEM INSTALLED IN GLASGOW ROYAL INFIRMARY

Data Preparation	2 ITT Creed Envoy Dataprinters
Input	Facit Paper Tape Reader 500/1000 cps
	IBM 1442 Card Read 300 cards/m
Output	Facit Paper Tape Punch 150 cps
	IBM 1442 Card Punch 80 cols/s
	IBM 1132 Line Printer 80–110 lpm
	IBM 1131 Console Printer 15 cps
Computer	IBM 1131 with 8K core store
	+ 2 disk drive backing store (total capacity approx. 1 million words)

All laboratory computer systems whether used off-line or on-line are used in Quality Control. This involves various straightforward statistical calculations, print out of results and an indication of whether or not they are within acceptable limits (Whitby, Mitchell, and Moss, 1967). In some on-line systems if excessive drift is detected or a control result is outwith limits an error signal is given and no further specimen results are printed.

Few systems, however, seem to employ the second-stage quality control which we have been doing since it was introduced in this laboratory several years ago by the late Dr. Eaton and Miss Gardner. In this system each current result is checked against previous results obtained from the same patient and rather frequent analytical and transcription errors are detected—in one short series we detected on average more than two errors a day. This system does not differ significantly from one which offers a cumulative report and we are at present proposing to do this by computer. The main problems are the adequacy of patient identification and the requirements for a fairly large backing store which should be preferably of the fast 'random access' type such as disk.

Our present computer system which was installed very recently is summarized in *Table V*.

We believe that this system will be sufficiently flexible to permit the investigation of two problems. The first is the examination of off-line data transmission between laboratories, thus offering computer facilities to small laboratories for which alone the installation cost of a computer would be unjustified. The power of our IBM 1130 installation is such that spare capacity will be available for this exercise. Although this has been successfully achieved in Uppsala (Hjelm, 1969), using an IBM 1130, with the 1080 Data Acquisition System and 1050 Data Transmission System, it does not seem to have been attempted in this country using the cheaper paper-tape-to-paper-tape systems. Whitby, Proffitt, and McMaster (1968) had some difficulties in using a central computer linked to the laboratory by teletypes and for this reason we have selected the more expensive Creed Envoy equipment. With the large population and distribution of hospitals in the Glasgow Area and Scottish Western Region (*Scottish Health Statistics*, 1969) it still seems essential to obtain experience in data transmission.

The second problem is related to developments in mechanized analysis. There are some 'discrete' systems under development which give the result directly as a single voltage and the trend with AutoAnalyser systems is towards so-called 'steady state' multi-channel systems which also give a single voltage for each result. Peak-picking software and the advantage of on-line operation may become obsolete unless the computer is used as a control unit (as with the AutoChemist) (Northam, 1969) or very rapid rates of analysis are achieved (as with the GEMSEC centrifuge system) (Anderson, 1969).

As the gap between programmable calculators and small computers is bridged I imagine the small computer will come to be regarded as a common and essential laboratory instrument and as hospital systems develop they will either use their own backing store or the hospital 'data bank'. The true costs of commercial time-sharing are too high for this to be considered as a realistic alternative despite its many attractions.

REFERENCES

ABERNETHY, M. H., BENTLEY, G. T., GARTELMANN, D., GRAY, P., OWEN, J. A., and QUAN SING, G. D. (1970), 'An Improved Computer Based, Multi-Channel System for Automatic Chemical Analysis', *Clinica chim. Acta*, **30**, 463.

ANDERSON, N. G. (1969), 'The Development of Automated Systems for Clinical and Research Use', *Ibid.*, **25**, 321.

BAIRD, H. W., GARFUNKEL, J. M. (1965), 'Electronic Data Processing of Medical Records', *New Engl. J. Med.*, **272**, 1211.

DAWSON, J. B., MILNER, R., and MAWSTON, D. (1969), 'A Simple Trace Reader With Digital Print-Out', *Analyst*, **94**, 912.

GRIFFITHS, P. D., and CARTER, N. W. (1969), 'On-Line Acquisition of the Output of AutoAnalysers', *J. clin. Path.*, **22**, 609.

HICKS, G. P., GIESCHEN, M. M., SLACK, W. V., and LARSON, F. C. (1966), 'Routine Use of a Small Digital Computer in the Clinical Laboratory', *J. Am. med. Ass.*, **196**, 973.

HJELM, M. (1969), 'The Handling and Processing of Data in a Clinical Biochemistry Laboratory', *Z. Klin. Chem. u. Klin. Biochem.*, **7**, 96.

KATONA, P. G., PAPPALARDO, A. N., MARBLE, C. W., BARNETT, G. O., and PASHBY, M. M. (1969), 'Automated Chemistry Laboratory: Application of a Novel Time-Shared Computer System', *Proc. Inst. Electrical and Electronic Eng.*, **57**, 2000.

NORTHAM, B. E. (1969), 'Discrete Analysis Systems', *J. clin. Path.*, **22**, Suppl. (Coll. Path.), 3, 42.

RAPPOPORT, A. E., GENNARO, W. D., and CONSTANDSE, W. J. (1968), 'Computer-Laboratory Link is Base of Hospital Information System', *Modern Hosp.*, **110**, 94.

SCOTTISH HEALTH STATISTICS, 1967 (1969), Edinburgh: H.M.S.O.

TILSTONE, W. J., and FLECK, A. (1970), 'Influence of Transcription Techniques on the Precision of AutoAnalyser Assays', *Proc. Nutr. Soc.*, **29**, 85.

WHITBY, L. G., MITCHELL, F. L., and MOSS, D. W. (1967), 'Quality Control in Routine Clinical Chemistry' in *Advances in Clinical Chemistry*, (Ed. BODANSKY, O., and STEWART, C. P.). Vol. **10**, 65. London: Academic.

— — PROFFITT, J., and McMASTER, R. S. (1968), 'Experience with Off-Line Processing by Computer of Chemical Laboratory Data', *Scott. med. J.*, **13**, 181.

— and SIMPSON, D. (1969), 'Experience with On-Line Computing in Clinical Chemistry', *J. clin. Path.*, **22**, Suppl. (Coll. Path.), 3, 107.

WHITEHEAD, T. P. (ed.) (1969), 'Automation and Data Processing in Pathology', *Ibid.*, **22** (Suppl.).

DISCUSSION

Question (Dr. A. W. Cull): Has the lecturer managed to solve the problem of infallible labelling of patients and specimens ?

Answer: No. In our work the first step is to check the compatibility of specimen and request form, and since they arrive in the laboratory in discrete batches from each ward (in plastic bags) this is usually straightforward. However, the problem of labelling and identification of the specimen in the ward does not seem to have received the attention it deserves. Within the laboratory the specimen and request form are linked by the accession number and only very rarely does confusion arise.

Comment (Dr. J. H. Mitchell): If one has a mechanically documentated system, then the hospital can produce a series of printed labels which can be put on specimens.

Answer: I think most hospitals will go on to addressing labels by mechanical means.

Question (Dr. A. W. Cull): Could you, please, comment on the value and usefulness of computerized information bearing in mind the immense number of tests done at hospitals.

Answer: A group in Toronto investigated this some years ago. They carried out a fixed large number of tests on all out-patients over a period even when only one investigation was requested, and later checked the results with the clinicians concerned. The reaction of the medical staff to anomalous results was interesting. For example, some recalled the patients for further investigation and others decided quite arbitrarily that the anomaly was due to laboratory error.

There have been suggestions recently that the optimum amount of data which can be scanned rapidly simultaneously and appreciated lies between 5 and 9 items.

Comment (D. Simpson): I would like to comment on the use of linear interpolation methods. Each point is accepted only if it lies within close pre-set limits so that the method does bear some comparison with the least squares or polynomial fits mentioned by Dr. Fleck.

SESSION 4

Chairman: Professor W. I. Card

*Le secret d'ennuyer est celui
de tout dire.*

VOLTAIRE

Computers in hospital administration

J. Emlyn Jones

THE popular concept of a hospital in the minds of the general public is to a considerable extent still that of Emergency Ward 10 or Dr. Kildare, according to the television channel watched and even those who have a more intimate association with hospitals, and amongst these I would include the members of the medical profession, often fail to appreciate how sophisticated in business as well as in technical issues a modern hospital has become. A modern hospital today is truly amongst the most complex business organizations existing in our modern society, demanding of its management all the techniques and abilities normally thought of as the perquisite of large industries and mammoth commercial undertakings. In manpower alone, the National Hospital Service in England is the direct employer of over $\frac{1}{2}$ million people of which slightly less than half relate to medical and nursing staff (*Table VI*). The scope for management in a manpower situation of such magnitude is self evident.

Patients enter hospital for a number of reasons, but primarily it is for medical and nursing care and attention. It is indicative of the present complex state of our hospital activities that if the services necessary to that patient's care are measured in terms of money, the purely medical and nursing portion forms the minor part of the overall cost. In 1970/71, the estimated revenue expenditure on hospital services in England within the National Health Service amounted to nearly £860 million (*Table VII*) of which two-thirds related to the remuneration of staff. Within this head

Table VI.—STAFF EMPLOYED IN THE NATIONAL HOSPITAL SERVICE IN
ENGLAND AT 30th SEPT., 1969

	Number	Per Cent
Medical and dental staff	21,817	4
Nursing and midwifery staff	231,469	44
Professional and technical staff connected with diagnosis and treatment (other than medical, dental and nursing)	32,058	6
Administrative and clerical staff (including architectural, surveying and engineering staff at R.H.B.'s)	46,556	9
Works maintenance, domestic, catering, and laundry, etc., staff	190,241	37
Totals	522,141	100

Table VII.—HOSPITAL SERVICE ESTIMATED REVENUE EXPENDITURE 1970–1
(ENGLAND ONLY)

	£M.	Per Cent	£M.	Per Cent
Central administration expenditure of boards and management committees			25·7	3·0
Hospital running expenses:				
Salaries and wages:				
Medical and dental	87·1	10·1		
Nursing	226·6	26·4		
Building and engineering	23·2	2·7		
Administrative and clerical	35·3	4·1		
Professional and technical	42·1	4·9		
Catering, domestic, portering, etc.	152·2	17·7		
			566·5	65·9
Provisions			47·8	5·6
Uniforms and clothing			6·2	0·7
Drugs, dressings, medical and surgical appliances			67·1	7·8
General services (lighting, heating, laundry, etc.)			41·8	4·9
Maintenance of buildings			21·9	2·6
Domestic repairs			10·5	1·2
All other expenses (net)			12·2	1·4
Other expenditure:				
(B.T.S., contractual arrangements, etc.)			13·2	1·5
Selective employment tax			46·4	5·4
Totals			859·3	100

the cost of the combined non-professional staff was broadly equal to the cost of the total nursing staff employed, and the wages of the domestic staff were indeed a larger total sum than the salaries and remuneration of the medical and dental staff of all grades. In the non-staff areas, the expenditure on food and textiles was very similar to the expenditure on drugs, dressings, and medical

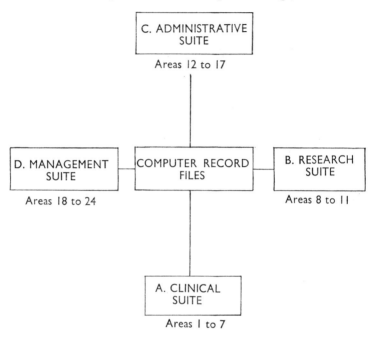

Fig. 32.—Integrated hospital computer application.

requisites. It is therefore not surprising that one of the most important areas of hospital activity is its administrative and management function, if administration has the responsibility for ensuring that the necessary hospital services are available to support the direct medical and nursing care.

The areas of administration and clinical function in hospitals do not readily lend themselves to rigid definition, as each of necessity must associate itself so closely with the other. With the introduction of computers and comprehensive data banks, it is likely that any previous distinction may become even more artificial. Consequently, in considering both the function and application of computers in the hospital service, whether in the administrative or clinical fields, it is as well first to identify those areas in which the computer could usefully be employed.

An integrated hospital computer application has been hypothesized by the Department of Health as comprising a number of suites, each suite covering a number of areas (*Fig.* 32, *Tables VIII–XI*). The areas have been included in the suite indicative

Table VIII.—A, CLINICAL AREAS

1. Patient screening	Tests, results, follow-up (e.g., cervical cytology)
2. Drugs and pharmacy	Requisitions, stock issues and receipts and records. Verified requests. Drug schedules
3. Laboratory services (biochemistry, haematology, bacteriology and histology)	Requests, specimen collection, results. Work load schedules
4. Therapeutic radiology	Radiation treatment, planning radiation protection
5. Operating theatre	Patient monitoring, pre-operation procedures. Staff availability, theatre demands, lists, and changes. Medical record display
6. E.C.G., E.E.G., and E.M.G.	Requests, appointments, analysis, results
7. Diagnostic radiology	Isotopes. Radiation protection. Requests, appointments, pre X-ray diets, results. Materials, receipts usage, stocks and ordering

Table IX.—B, RESEARCH AREAS

8. Ad hoc research	E.g., morbidity and epidemiology
9. Research statistics	Standard statistical techniques for quality control and applied research
10. Operational research	Mathematical investigation of managerial, administrative and medical problems
11. Diagnosis	Hospital activity analysis, diagnostic records and indices, routine diagnostic aid

of their primary purpose, although in many instances the areas can extend into two or more suites. Neither the suites nor the areas are necessarily exclusive but from this hypothesis it is a reasonable inference that the more immediate problem is to determine which areas should receive priority consideration in the introduction of computers and a number of studies and applications are currently being undertaken into certain of these areas, some studies being more advanced than others. In the short time available to me I should like to touch on the use of computers in the administrative and management areas with which I have been personally concerned and which in the main are operational today. But in doing so, I propose to draw my main distinction between computer systems rather than hospital functional activities.

Computing systems are classified in a variety of ways, ranging from their functional purpose to the methodology involved. The classification which seems to be most appropriate to the hospital administrative service is that which distinguishes between:—

    a. Information processing systems,

    b. Recall systems, and

    c. Control systems.

Table X.—C, ADMINISTRATIVE AREAS

12. Transport scheduling	Transport lists, availability, demands, allocations
13. Catering	Menu planning, special diets, supplies, food price variation
14. Ward and theatre management	Bed state, operating lists, nurse allocation, laboratory tests, treatments, diets, drugs, patient monitoring
15. Medical records	Data to and from all other functions of the administrative and clinical suits and to the management and research suites
16. In-patients	Register, waiting list, admissions, discharges and letters to general practitioners
17. Out-patients	Waiting lists, appointments, medical staff availability, clinic lists, attendances, discharge letters to general practitioners

Table XI.—D, MANAGEMENT AREAS

18. Paymaster and stewardship functions	Payroll, paybills, stores, accounting records, annual statements
19. Management accounting	Cash allocations and expenditure department costing, current and future budgeting
20. Management statistics	Hospital activity analysis, resources allocation
21. Costing	Illness, therapy, drugs, catering
22. Personnel	Manpower data, planning, recruitment needs, allocation
23. Supplies	Stock levels, usage analysis
24. Planning, construction, engineering	Critical path analysis, bills of quantities, resource allocation and scheduling. Commissioning

Most of the applications in the service, both current and prospective, have hitherto fallen within the first two, although increasingly attention is being directed towards the last of these categories.

An information processing system in this context is one that collects, analyses, and processes information to the requirement of the user, and within the Health Service as in other organizations the first use of computers was in this field as applied to accounting functions. It is increasingly popular these days to disparage the use of computers for what is termed 'the commercial application' by which the critics refer to the production of payrolls, accounting records and paybill schedules. But so far as the National Health Service is concerned, these are the very areas in which computers have been successful and which now are in general use by most hospital authorities.

The production of a payroll, whether it be in Industry or Public Service with all its associated schedules and accounting, is by no means a simple task in these days of vigorous wage negotiation and social taxation. It is perhaps because the National Health Service lacks the discipline of a measurable end product that the wage structures of the staff employed in hospitals have become as complex and as illogical as any to be found elsewhere.

Under the National Health Service Acts all officers employed in the Service are officers of the Regional Boards or Boards of Governors. Nevertheless, in practice the direct employing authorities, i.e., Regional Boards, Boards of Governors, and Hospital Management Committees are responsible for the employment of their staffs and the calculations and payment of their salaries and wages. Instead, therefore, of a relatively small number of paying authorities (14 Regional Hospital Boards and 35 Boards of Governors) in England, there are in fact 348 hospital authorities of one order or another, all of whom could and at one time did, operate their own system of wage calculation and produce their own payrolls, subject only to the limitation of the terms and conditions of service that had been agreed nationally. This was both a wasteful and expensive utilization of manpower and with the increasing complexity of pay conditions and the developing difficulty of training and retaining competent pay staff, the advent of computers made alternative methods attractive.

My own region (Manchester) today deals with 100,000 employees through its computer system, half of whom are paid at weekly intervals and the other half at monthly intervals. The pay scales appropriate to these 100,000 staff number nearly 1000, the majority of which can have incremental pay additions ranging from 3 to 15. In addition, of course, ancillary staff are paid according to hours actually worked at appropriate hourly rates.

One of the first requirements of a pay information system is to give the person being paid adequate details of his remuneration and it is invariable practice today to do this through a pay notification slip. It is an important part of management/labour relationships that the employee be given such information as is necessary for him to check his gross and net earnings, but with the additional facilities now demanded of employers there is a continuing conflict between information asked for by the employee and the often practical as well as economic burden placed on the employer. Currently our own notification slip (*Fig.* 33) provides 26 items of pay make-up as well as information on pay entitlement, but increasing and expanding demands keep this format in a continuous state of review.

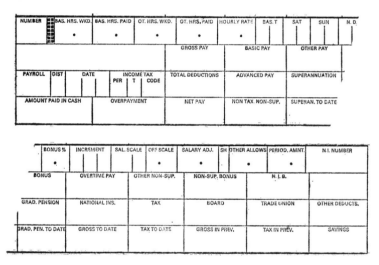

Fig. 33.—Notification slip.

The necessary calculation and notification at individual level of gross pay entitlements, additions, deductions and net amounts payable are not, however, the only requirement of a payroll system. The subsequent processes carried out depend on management's requirements and in our own case, every payroll supplies considerable information in addition to the individual pay notification.

The spin offs of the computer system include the control and discharge of the compulsory functions placed on the employer, such as tax collection under P.A.Y.E., graduated pension, S.E.T., and National Insurance deductions under the respective statutory provisions, and any other that may be required, as well as similar services of a non-statutory nature, such as the collection and accounting for trade union subscriptions, savings scheme, collection of charges, etc., which seem to be growing in importance in the employer/employee relationship. In all, 301 totals (*Table XII*)

Table XII.—Payroll Final Totals

1. Totals for current pay period:—
   a. Basic pay
   b. Overtime pay
   c. National insurance benefit deducted
   d. Gross pay entitlement
   e. Tax deducted under P.A.Y.E.
   f. Graduated pension deducted
   g. Superannuation contribution deducted
   h. National insurance contribution deducted
   i. Payment for board and lodging
   j. Recovery of overpayments
   k. Recovery of advance payment
   l. Any other deductions
   m. Net pay entitlement
   n. Net pay actually paid
2. Cumulative information relative to previous and this employment on gross pay and tax.
3. Current period and cumulative information on employer's liability for superannuation, graduated pension, national insurance, S.E.T., etc.
4. Analysis of other deductions over 99 heads. (Note: 29 refer to Trade Union Subscriptions).
5. Coinage analysis over 8 elements for up to 5 distribution points.
6. National insurance stamp analysis over 19 values sub-divided between the four contribution years.
7. Control totals on staff variations and numbers paid.
   Number of separate totals printed = 301.

supported by the necessary detail are available to management, the need for a large number of which in the National Health Service has been imposed by the central authority either in its function as national hospital authority or as central government.

Similar information processing systems have been developed in the expenditure/stores areas wherein materials, commitments, and services are paid for, accounted for and analysed in accordance with the requirements of the Service. Spin offs from these areas which have as their first responsibility the stewardship aspect lead into the costing and functional management fields.

Information processing systems are by no means limited to commercial or accounting applications. One of the areas that has taken advantage of this approach is the quantity surveying section of the Architect's Department of the Board, who over the last five years have developed and currently use a computer programme for the preparation of bills of quantities, based upon the library/look-up technique. But probably the most used non-commercial application of this system is the development of the hospital statistical service based on patient statistics and known as Hospital Activity Analysis (H.A.A.). The main purpose of Hospital Activity Analysis is to provide clinicians and administrators at all levels with information relating to patient activities under which details of individual patients are brought together for summation and analyses: these include clinical information relating to diagnosis and operations and patient characteristics such as sex, marital status, and area of residence. Administrative information about admission, stay and discharge is also included. The full information included in this analysis comprises 25 items (*Table XIII*).

Analyses are extracted from the data banks according to the needs of the users, either in the form of routine schedules or by way of ad hoc enquiries. The present routine analyses in the Manchester region comprise 12 tables (*Table XIV*), the first 6 of which cover predominantly the admission, stay, and discharge functions, and the next 6 matters of more clinical and research interest.

The ad hoc enquiries are usually of a research nature and are generally restricted to an individual interest.

The development of H.A.A. has been going on now for some years and there is not unexpectedly an uneven pattern of development over the country as a whole. In some regions up to 100 per cent of the eligible discharges fall within the ambit of the scheme, whereas in other regions the scheme is in a comparatively early stage of development. In the Manchester region about 50 per cent of the non-psychiatric hospitals are currently participating, representing approximately 220,000 patient records. Within the next 18 months the remainder will be taken on, by which time 400,000 patient records will be processed annually. As each patient record provides for 160 alpha/numer characters the quantities of data (45 million characters annually on average) as well as the accessibility of data are major problems.

But the collection and processing of mass information are not the only benefits computers can bring to administrative functions.

Much of our time and effort is involved in recall procedures—that is bringing back selective pieces of information—and developments have been proceeding with the use of computers for this purpose. In my own region particularly we have developed two such applications, both of which are now operational.

Table XIII.—Hospital Activity Analysis
Patient Information

1. Hospital	14. Date of admission
2. Unit No.	15. Disposal
3. Sex	16. Date of discharge
4. Address code	17. Place of accident
5. Date of birth	18. Previous pregnancies
6. Place of birth	19. Principal diagnosis
7. Marital status	20. Underlying cause
8. Category of patient	21. Other relevant conditions
9. Source of admission	22. Visits to theatre
10. Date on waiting list	23. Days before operation
11. Consultant	24. Operation code 1
12. Specialty	25. Operation code 2
13. Ward	

Table XIV.—Routine Analysis Provided by H.A.A.

Quarterly
1. By hospital ward and consultant:—
     a. Source of admission
     b. Number of days before operation
2. By hospital, specialty and consultant:—
     a. Average length of stay
     b. Discharges and deaths
3. By emergency admissions:—
     a. As percentage of total admissions by specialty
4. By consultant:—
     a. Time spent on waiting list
5. Incidence of malignant cancer, by Unit No. and hospital
6. Diagnostic analysis of general medical and general surgical emergencies
7. Analysis of:—
     a. Squints, cataracts, corneal grafts, etc.
     b. Abortions
     c. Orthopaedic patients
Annually
     Extraction of H.I.P.E. records for General Register Office.

In 1963, the then Minister of Health decided to make cytological screening for cervical cancer available to all women at risk and hospital authorities were urged to provide the necessary facilities adequate to screen the appropriate classes of patients at specified intervals. The patient class has been extended and the frequency increased since those early days.

The scheme requires the taking of smears, the provision of laboratory facilities, the registration and recording of patient information, a follow-up and recall procedure, and a fee payment to general practitioners. Since 1963, the service in the Manchester region has been centred on the Christie Hospital and Holt Radium Institute under the direction of Dr. R. Yule, who have been providing the necessary laboratory facilities and maintaining the appropriate patient records. By 1968, approximately 150,000 cytology records were being maintained at the hospital in manual card files and this file was increasing at the rate of 25,000 new patients per year. It was therefore decided to transfer the record keeping, the recall procedure and the general practitioner's fee payment to a computer system which has now been done.

As always, one of the greatest difficulties in any patient information system is the positive identification of the patient and, in the then absence of a unique patient number, one had to be created based on the details of surname, maiden name, and birth. The patient record has had to be constructed in variable length form to provide narrative details of the patient, e.g., name, address, birth, etc., as well as the details of the results of a maximum twelve smears.

Validation of information and up-dating the main file with details of new smears, new patients, etc., currently takes place fortnightly and output consists of fortnightly call-up letters, annual payment of doctors' fees and such statistical information as is requested by the hospital unit.

Because the system is not 'on line' the hospital is required to maintain a patient index card file which is kept up to date by the computer producing new index cards when up-dating the computer main file, but a future development may well be a direct 'on line' service between the hospital and the computer centre.

Call-up letters are produced fortnightly for the following categories of patients:—

> 10 per cent of those eligible for 3-monthly call-up
> 10 per cent of those eligible for 1-yearly call-up
> 10 per cent of those eligible for 2-yearly call-up
> 100 per cent of those eligible for 3-yearly call-up

Patients are eligible for recall purposes once they have had a normal smear read at the regional cytology laboratory. Each patient is only recalled once for research purposes but will be automatically recalled after three years have elapsed from the date of her last normal smear. If no response is received within a specified time of recall—currently eight weeks—a reminder letter is produced.

The first recall procedure by computer took place last July and during the first year's operation, 110,000 recall letters at the rate of 4400 per fortnight are expected to be produced. These numbers are based on an existing main file of 210,000 patient records but as this is a cumulative process and the main file is now expected to increase by 40,000/50,000 new patients per annum, an increasingly heavy burden of recall is anticipated and will have to be faced.

Smears are of course being received from several sources and in order to authorize the appropriate fee payment an identification of the source is necessary. Currently the participants comprise 1400 General Practitioners, 75 Local Health Authorities, 75 Family Planning Associations, and 3 hospitals, and a computer programme has been developed which identifies the smear taken by each general practitioner entitled to a fee payment, computes the sum due, and prepared a summary of the smears taken, together with a cheque for the appropriate amount.

As the computer scheme is relatively of recent origin, the statistical output has still to be developed to any extent and as yet only an analysis of smears taken by local authorities over the fifteen months to March, 1970, has been extracted. As the recall procedures swing in full operation, there is little doubt that extended analyses will become a routine function within the system.

Another somewhat similar application of computers to a recall situation is the recently developed donor call-up procedure in the Blood Transfusion Service. As probably all of you know, the Blood Transfusion Service is an organization administered by Regional Hospital Boards for the collection, processing, and distribution of blood for the use of hospital patients. Blood is obtained from voluntary donors enrolled from the public at large and listed on regional blood donor panels. Because of personal factors the donation rate of people called is less than 50 per cent, i.e., of every two donors asked to attend a session to give blood, on average slightly less than one actually gives blood. The aim of the administration, of course, is to obtain the greatest donation of blood from the least number of donors called and it was because the donation rate had been dropping for some years that a study was made as to whether improvements could be effected in the call-up procedures of the Blood Transfusion Service if the facilities of a computer were available.

A system was therefore developed to select donors from a central data bank and schedule their attendance at donor sessions according to predetermined selection priorities and current donor data continuously maintained in the record.

The system is based on the completion of a session slip which acts as a dual purpose document—as input to the system for the creation or amendment of donors' records and as output of the system for session information and control. Donor selection and scheduling take place within parameters determined by the Blood Transfusion Service organization.

The main file contains three types of record:—

1. Donor record in registration number order within panel.
2. Panel status records giving information on current and prospective availability of donor within the panel.
3. Statistical records relating to attendances at sessions, response ratios, etc.

Output data is available for four main purposes:—

1. For session control and registration.
2. For office use through panel status tables, selection schedules, individual call-up notices, and full donor record print-outs.
3. For laboratory use giving the medical and technical information required by that department.
4. Statistical breakdown as required.

Up-date and donor extract programmes are run daily and session schedules produced 3 weeks before each session. Call-up documents (postcards) are produced 14 days before the session date and final slips and check list made available 1 day before the session at which the donors are scheduled to attend. Panel status tables are printed out weekly or as required. Laboratory information is notified the morning following the session and statistical information is supplied at intervals as required by the Blood Transfusion Service administration.

Although at present the computer application is restricted to the calling-up of donors and the maintenance of their records, the main advantage of the system is its flexibility and development potential, particularly in the fields of call-up rationalization and blood bank inventory control.

There are other areas in which information systems, recall procedures or a combination of both are being applied or developed. To mention only a further few, waiting lists, catering functions, and resource allocations are all the subject of present experimentation and study in a computer context. But all these applications have one thing in common—the collection of masses of data in a central record for a limited functional use. But there is now a rapidly expanding realization that information contained in data banks should not be limited to their initial purpose. Much of the payroll data currently used for the payment of personal remuneration could form the base of a manpower planning application incorporating recruitment, labour allocations, environmental studies and similar issues. Accounting systems should incorporate cost analyses, budgeting procedures, resource benefit assessments, etc. Stores accounting should be a support as well as a check of a supplies and purchasing system. Even clinical areas cannot remain free from the impact of hospital activity analysis, patient appointment schedules, etc.

If we accept that one of the essential functions of administration is to obtain the greatest benefit from the use of available resources, whether this benefit is measured in monetary terms or in patient services, we must also accept that the use of sophisticated management techniques will grow in the National Health Service. There is also little doubt that in order to apply these management techniques the utilization of computers and similar modern aids will be necessary. Public services generally, including the hospital service have been in the forefront in the application of mechanical systems including computers to accounting functions. The further extension of computers to the other administrative fields in the National Health Service has not advanced as quickly as some of us had hoped, but the fairly near future will, through the adoption of these proved techniques, show a rapid development of the use of computers in the hitherto excluded areas, thus leading to the more efficient management of our hospitals and to the benefit of the patients requiring our services.

DISCUSSION

Question: Are nurse allocations made on computers in Manchester ?

Answer: A feasibility study was undertaken by the Tavistock Institute on behalf of the Manchester Board into a computer allocation system but their recommendation was that an assistant matron could do this as well. I understand that Dr. Clark of the University of Manchester Medical Computing Centre has undertaken some studies here; I believe that some relevant work has also been done by Mr. James at Liverpool, and by Dr. Barr at the Oxford Regional Hospital Board. None of these studies to my knowledge has become fully operational.

Question: Has any time study been done ?

Answer: No.

Computers in the assessment of medical students

Bernard Lennox and Agnes A. C. Wallace

THE subject is somewhat marginal to the present conference, for essentially it is part of educational technology rather than medicine: but there are several reasons for including it. Most of the medicals who have been active in the computer fields are on the staff of medical schools, and have a necessary interest in examinations. A surprising amount of the pioneer work on examination techniques in this country at the university level, both in the introduction of multiple choice methods and in their machine marking, has occurred in the medical faculties, who have often seemed at least as interested in the subject as the professional educationalists. It has the advantage that it presents from the computer point of view a relatively straightforward problem in data handling, rather than computation, and it is therefore a useful test situation for some of the problems involved at one level in the medical field. And finally, if properly handled, it can be useful propaganda to the medical students on the possibilities of computing.

All we can speak of from personal experience is the use of computers in marking multiple-choice questions (M.C.Q.), and most of our time will be spent on that, with some emphasis on the possibilities of setting up a unit to service M.C.Q. on a national scale. But it may be worth a reminder that this is far from being the only application which could be discussed.

STUDENT RECORDS

This relatively mundane matter ought to be accepted as part of assessment: it is no use examining a student if you cannot efficiently record and recall and if possible analyse the results. Some kind of activity of this kind is under way in most universities, and a few medical faculties have schemes of their own. Glasgow University has a rather skeletal system of computerized records dealing with matriculation, fees, and class lists, and this is slowly expanding.

In the medical faculty we have begun work on a system for dealing with candidates for admission, with the object in the first place of keeping track of the large number of unconditional and conditional offers outstanding and producing a best estimate of the number of actual admissions they represent, and ultimately of undertaking a thorough analysis of selection criteria. We have also been asked by the faculty to look into the possibility of a more thorough-going computerization of student records right through the course. We are by no means certain whether it will be worth while: one would expect most people to be somewhat daunted by the prospect of a systems analysis of the Dean's office.

A good deal that is worth while might be done, however, in the recording of examination results. Our present methods of dealing with the inter-relationships of different examinations are very crude, whether by way of finding an index of total achievement over the whole course, or detecting correlations between different examinations. But it could be made easier. Marks might be converted to standard deviations above and below the mean for each examination, which would eliminate the effects of the considerable variation between examinations not only in standard (which is obvious from the fail rate) but also in scatter. It ought also to be possible, by comparing the overall results for each examination over successive years, to bring to light variations in marking standards from year to year. There are plenty of other functions of a computerized student record system that would be of value in any assessment procedure, and as we move further in the direction of continuous assessment (or at least less discontinuous assessment, for we hope that the state of almost daily testing that some envisage will never be reached) its usefulness will increase.

There is, of course, the much more exciting field of simulation. There are all sorts of ways in which the computer can pretend to be a patient for the student to practise on, at all levels, from using a teleprinter to respond to the right questions with the gist of a clinical history, to actuating a dummy responding to anaesthesia. Mostly these have been thought of purely as teaching machines, but they could equally be used for examination. A student's ability to progress through a session of programmed learning with a minimum of wrong turnings is after all excellent evidence of good progress in the subject, and computer control of the process should make it all the easier to assess his standing. There seems little doubt that all this is practicable; one must doubt only, as with so many computer schemes, whether it is worth the cost—not only the computer cost, both for hardware and software, but the cost of the immense amount of medical teachers' time needed to devise the simulations. For the present, we should regard this as a subject for research, but it could very well loom very large in the future.

M.C.Q.

FORMATS

It is useful first to consider what kind of question one may be asked to mark. The name 'multiple-choice-question' should be confined to those in which the candidate is offered a choice of two or more answers to a given question, and must choose the one among them which the examiner has decided beforehand is the only correct response. In general it is sound policy to keep the format as simple as possible. We want particularly to make the point that simplicity of structure of the examination paper, which makes computerization so much easier, makes in fact for a better examination in any case. In general, only two basic formats have any great currency in this country. Most undergraduate examinations use the one-from-five:—

Gastric ulcers occur in which one of the following?
A. Oesophagus   B. Stomach   C. Duodenum   D. Jejunum   E. Ileum.

One-from-four is an unimportant variant of this. Basically similar, however different it appears at first sight, is the grouped M.C.Q.:—

For each of the conditions on the left, indicate the most common site from those on the right:—

1.	Amoebic dysentery	A.	Oesophagus
2.	Argentaffinoma	B.	Stomach
3.	Atrophic gastritis	C.	Duodenum
4.	Gastric ulcer	D.	Ileum
5.	Squamous carcinoma	E.	Jejunum
		F.	Appendix
		G.	Colon.

This is a labour-saving device for the examiner, but it introduces a minor problem in computerization, in that it increases the number of possible answers which have to be offered. Most programs can deal with it, but simple ones such as our own cannot, and we have adopted as a temporary expedient a kind of mini grouped

M.C.Q. in which we ask three questions and offer the same five possible answers for each of them. It is a satisfactory format only if one occasionally uses the same answer twice in one group (having of course warned the examinee that one may do so), so that if he knows the answers to two questions out of the three he cannot count on having narrowed the choice for the third down to the three unused possible answers.

The other main variety is the true/false. This is in fact a one-from-two, but it is nearly always presented as the true/false form—

Gastric ulcers occur in the stomach: true or false ?

This is the type most used in postgraduate examinations, and appears there mostly in a rather odd format:—

Peptic ulcers occur in:—
A. Oesophagus   B. Stomach   C. Duodenum   D. Jejunum   E. Ileum.

This looks like a one-from-five with the only-one-right-answer restriction removed, but it is of course a series of five independent true/falses—Peptic ulcers occur in the oesophagus—true/false ?, in the stomach—true/false ?, etc. (The example is not a very good question as it stands, by the way: is a peptic ulcer in a Meckel diverticulum 'in' the ileum or not ?)

Recognition of this format as a true-false variant makes computer marking much easier, for to treat them in any other way means the introduction of considerably more complex scoring systems, none of which is wholly satisfactory. It ought also to make for greater flexibility in setting: examiners in most of the Colleges seem still to be hypnotized by this grouping into fives, which often means taking a subject that is worth two or three items and padding it out. Examiners ought to be encouraged to shorten or occasionally lengthen the groups to match the size of the subject, and it is worth making sure that the computer programs, as well as such things as the design of answer sheets and even the mode of numbering of the questions, are not so inflexible as to prevent this.

SCORING

This is a large subject, but only some of the arguments are relevant here. Again there is everything to be said for simplicity: it is possible with a computer to apply all sorts of complicated weightings and the like, but the temptation should be resisted unless you are prepared to lay on at the same time a completely thought out research plan to evaluate your ideas, and still resisted fairly firmly even if you are. Each question should be worth one mark for a right answer: a standard countermark should be subtracted for each wrong answer, high enough to discourage guessing: and the candidate should be permitted to make a nil return to a question for which he does not know the answer—that is to say he ought not to be forced to guess. Also the candidate should be told what the scoring system is, and if he is inexperienced care should be taken to ensure that he understands its implications. All this will be balm to your programmer, unless he is anxious to make difficulties for himself.

Unless for research purposes (and then only if you know quite clearly what the object of your research is) there is no need to ask for anything very complicated in the way of output. A single list of candidates in alphaaetical (or other convenient) order, showing the score of each, is the main thing. It may be necessary to divide the paper up into sections, but there is not much profit if the divisions are small. It is easy and often helpful to provide a second list in order of score, as a guide to distribution and a help in determining any cut-off points. It may be worth calculating a mean and standard deviation at this stage, and there may be circumstances in which it is worth showing all scores in terms of standard deviations above and below the mean.

It is also essential to analyse the questions; indeed, except for very large examinations, there is little point in computerization unless one does this. But this need not be elaborate. One needs basically three pieces of information about each question:—

1. Its difficulty, best measured as an easiness index—the percentage of the maximum possible score on that question obtained by all the candidates together.

2. A discrimination index, measuring ability to separate good students from bad. There are many ways of calculating this, but none is wholly satisfactory, and the relatively simple ϕ coefficient (Hubbard and Clemans, 1961) suffices. It is unwise to read discrimination indices too literally: the causes of a low score are diverse, and by no means all of them indicate a poor question.

3. A simple tabulation of the number of candidates who have responded to each of the possible answers, and of the number who have avoided it altogether—the most useful feed-back to teachers especially.

None of these present any special difficulty in programming and they give all the information needed for all ordinary purposes.

SETTING STANDARDS

This worries people more than it need. Of course it is certainly possible to standardize standards, if one might be permitted the expression; it is for instance possible, by repeating questions, to compare the performance of one cohort of students with the next, or to compare classes in one place with those elsewhere. And, of course, a big organization with extensive facilities for computer analysis could do this very effectively. But the people who worry most are those just beginning to use the method. What usually happens is that they set a paper with great care and labour, and it proves too hard, and they find that if they apply their normal pass standard they fail twice as many candidates as usual. With experience, and without any elaborate analysis, most people soon find that it is easier than one might expect to achieve a roughly adequate level. But in any case, even with complete beginners setting the paper, provided they have a modicum of insight into the sort of thing their students can be expected to know, what the M.C.Q. paper will always do with considerable reliability is to put the students in the right order. One must realize that at this stage it will do no more, and one must rely on other elements in the examination to decide the pass or fail level.

This is a single aspect of a general point about such examinations: that while M.C.Q. are the most reliable single method of examination, a good examination should use as many different techniques as the circumstances permit. All the examiners in postgraduate examinations and the like, where most of the candidates are unknown to them, and external examiners in internal examinations, ought to spend as much of their time as possible in weighing up as many individual candidates as possible by methods involving personal contact. They may be wildly out in assessment of individual candidates (and in that case the evidence of a good M.C.Q. should probably weigh more than that of an oral) but in their judgement of the performance of the group as a whole, in their decision as to roughly how many are well enough prepared to go on to whatever next stage of their career is at stake, the consensus of a group of conscientious examiners is not often far out. This principle, the ultimate responsibility of examiners in contact with the candidates for the setting of standards, is one we ought never to forget. We can mechanize, computerize, dehumanize the examinations as much as we like, and the results, in terms of justice to the individual candidate, may be all to the good. But in the long run there must remain a human responsibility for the decision as to whether, as a group, the successful candidates are adequately prepared for whatever lies ahead of them. Even here, adequate follow-up of the subsequent careers of the candidates is a thing which would be very valuable for examiners who want to check the validity of their hunches, and computerized records might help here, but that only takes the illustration a stage further: one can delegate the donkey work to a machine, but not the responsibility.

THE COMPUTER INPUT

All the skilled work of an M.C.Q. paper occurs before the examination, when the examiners set the paper and decide the marking scheme. Everything thereafter ought to be purely mechanical. But of course the mechanism needs to be well engineered. Even with hand marking, there is a good deal to be learned about the design of answer sheets and the like. With computer marking, one comes up at once against the problem of getting the data into the computer—a classic data-handling situation. One has to have a system that can be operated by large numbers of operators totally without previous experience (though this is mitigated by above-average intelligence and a reasonable degree of motivation) and with an error rate that need not be o per cent but certainly should not be above 2 per cent for any one candidate (one should not count on an overall error rate of much under 5 per cent in any examination, but clearly even this could not be attained if arithmetical errors approaching that level had to be included).

The possible methods we have described in more detail elsewhere (Lennox and Wallace, 1970): they can be summarized as follows:—

1. Professional hand-punching. The candidate fills in conventional answer sheets by hand, and these are handed to punch operators who prepare either cards or tape from them in the usual manner. This is a relatively slow and expensive method, but if appropriate facilities are available at the right time and place, it can be both less slow and less expensive than one might suppose. It is more attractive to the Colleges, which can afford it, than to undergraduate departments, which have usually enough junior staff not to find hand marking too much of a burden. But it is not likely to survive where more direct methods are available.

2. Hole-poking. In this group of techniques the answer sheet is made of thin cardboard which has been pre-stamped in such a manner that holes of the right size and shape can readily be poked out in the correct position with a special stylus: the candidate has only to decide in which of the possible positions to poke out his hole for each question. In the usual form of this technique (such as the Portapunch) one ends up with a card like an ordinary Hollerith punch card, which can serve as a computer input with an ordinary card-reader. They are relatively cheap and require a minimum of ancillary apparatus. There are machines at about the £200 level which will count holes automatically, making scoring easy, though they are no help for question analysis. In practice, however, the cards are fiddly to use and surprisingly noisy in a large class, and they do not seem to be popular with students.

A variant pioneered by our own department of Medicine (Lever, Harden, Wilson and Jolley, 1970) is the use of very much larger cards of a type designed for feature card systems. They are much easier for the candidate to handle, and one card is sufficient for the great majority of examinations. Their main disadvantage up to the present has been the impossibility of using them for direct computer input, but a new machine has just arrived on the market which can transfer data from feature cards onto punched tape, and this will obviously change the position: our department of Medicine hope to be reporting on its usefulness.

3. Mark-sense card-punching. The method which has been most used in this country (Harris and Buckley-Sharp, 1968, 1970; Flinn, 1970), and which we have adopted ourselves (Lennox and Wallace, 1970), is the fully mechanized but two-stage process that uses a mark-sense card punch. In this the candidate makes pencil marks in prescribed spaces on a Hollerith type card, and the cards are fed into a punch with a reading head (which may be electromechanical—using the conductivity of graphite—or optical), and a hole is punched corresponding to each properly made mark. The cards are again fed into the card-reader of a computer. The method certainly works, and seems quite popular with students, though obviously they need careful instruction beforehand and supervision during the examination if they are to make their marks properly. The punches cost two or three thousand pounds, most of which goes on the punch mechanism which can be used for many other purposes, and they are fairly generally available. One suffers from being dependent on the functioning of two machines,

the punch and the computer, but so long as the punch works one can hand-score relatively easily by the use of masks—an advantage the method shares with the preceding technique.

4. Mark-sense tape punching. There are machines which read mark-sense documents and produce paper tape which can be used as a computer input. The Motorola is available in card-reading or sheet-reading forms and costs only a relatively few thousand pounds, but we know of no-one using it for this purpose in this country. The Lector is much bigger and faster, and needs skilled handling, but it certainly can be made to work (Gibbons and Wood, 1970; Anderson, 1970). We very nearly succeeded in being first to make it work for scoring M.C.Q. (Lennox and Duff, 1966), but were a little premature.

5. Mark sensing with direct input to computer. The Motorola could probably be used in this way, though it is probably too slow for this to be an economic system. The ICL Universal Document Transport is probably the best available prospect: it certainly is a machine that works, but it costs some £20,000 and can only be used on-line to a fairly substantial computer, so it is hardly attractive to the average user.

6. Two other possibilities may be worth mentioning. Magnetic ink pencils can be used for mark sensing (Ives, 1970) and would have some advantages; but the machines to read them are, we believe, no longer available. Optical character readers seem to be emerging at last into the sphere of practical techniques, at least to read standard type faces, and it might just prove possible to exploit this in some way in the future, though it is by no means obvious how.

COMPUTING THE RESULTS

The processing of the data, once they have been converted to a computer-readable form, is a very straightforward piece of pro-gramming, and what problems there are chiefly relate to saving computer time for a program that is likely to be used many times. It is obviously best to use a computer in which all the data can be stored at once on fast store, i.e., the number of available words of core or disk store should be greater than the number of candidates multiplied by the number of items on the paper—but there are no other constraints on the type of computer used. As so often, the main necessity is that the user should be able to define his requirements exactly, and there should be little excuse for failing to do that in this field.

Our original attempt in 1965 to devise a system ran into trouble chiefly with the conversion of data from the Lector tape output to the KDF9, but we have had no difficulty with our present program. It has been kept simple, chiefly as a matter of principle, but partly so as not to commit the University to any special format at this early stage, and partly because we are expecting soon to replace our present computer with something larger. We have used the Middlesex Hospital mark-sense cards (Harris and Buckley-Sharp, 1968), and the program is written in Egdon Algol. It has proved a surprisingly painless exercise, and our students have accepted the innovation with very few complaints and with a good deal of interest.

PROSPECTS

The use of M.C.Q. in medical schools in this country is still very patchy, but steadily increasing. Some use is made of them by more than half the undergraduate departments of pathology in the country, and we know of no medical school which is not using them at all. The use of computers in scoring is naturally less widespread, but is also increasing: most schools have at least made some experiments in this direction (Lennox and Lever, 1970). At least three centres (Middlesex Hospital, Newcastle, and Birmingham) operate successful marking services on an almost commercial basis for those who cannot do their own. There is certainly no lack of fully operational systems.

On the postgraduate side the Royal College of Physicians, London, were the pioneers (Owen, Robson, Sanderson, Smart, and Stokes, 1967) in a system that now embraces all the physicians' Colleges. The Royal College of Pathologists has also been active, using the Birmingham machine. The Glasgow College was the first to introduce M.C.Q. into the Primary Surgical Fellowship, but is still using hand marking: they have now completely abandoned essay questions, a change which has obviously been very popular with candidates. The Dublin College of Surgeons has just introduced M.C.Q., and has used a local bureau for computer marking from the outset.

It has been often suggested that this widespread but largely un-co-ordinated activity is wasteful, and that some kind of central organization should be set up. The Colleges were most active in promoting co-operation, and in July, 1969, a conference of Colleges and Medical Schools was held at the Royal College of Physicians,

London, at which it was agreed that a real need existed for such a service, and the Association for the Study of Medical Education (A.S.M.E.) was asked to prepare detailed proposals. A working party was set up by A.S.M.E. and has prepared a report which is to be submitted to a second conference of the same interested parties in the near future. Obviously one cannot anticipate the report in any detail, but it seems reasonable to mention one or two considerations that might be expected to seem obvious to anyone who gave the matter the careful consideration required of the working party.

NEEDS OF A CENTRAL MEDICAL EXAMINATIONS SERVICE

It is conceivable that such a service could be paid for by some central body such as the University Grant Committee on the basis that it was saving university departments so much staff time that this was to the benefit of university finance in general. But even if it were, it is likely that it would be run on at least some such pseudo-commercial basis as the Edinburgh Regional Computer Service, which charges for its services even if the money merely goes from one drawer to another of the same till—or perhaps one should update one's metaphor and say from one file to another of the same computer. One has to think of a service which at least in principle is charging a realistic price for its services and paying its way.

There is not much point in running a shoe-string service such as that provided by the three places already functioning. These use the space and staff and computing facilities of their universities or medical schools. They are able to pay for some of what they use, but are not really commercially viable. They manage some research, but only by using the spare time of their part-time medical managers. It might be possible to function by building up a unit of this type, or by reinforcing one or more of the existing units, but clearly what was envisaged by the original conference was something independent and self-supporting and on an altogether more ambitious scale.

Unfortunately once one begins to estimate the needs of such a self-standing unit, they begin to look formidable. It would need at least three fairly senior full-time non-medicals—a secretary, manager, and a research-and-development man who would need to know a lot about computing. They would need secretarial and programming staff. They would need either a good deal of equipment, including a computer which would need to be a good deal more than a bare PDP8, or free access by terminal to a big machine. They would need premises which would not be too isolated and would probably need to be in London. And while no doubt the great majority of the many medicals who would be involved in one way or another would be able to give their services free, there would almost certainly need to be a nucleus of medicals, including the director, who received some payment for part-time services. It all begins to add up to a great deal of money—not six figures per annum, perhaps, but heading in that direction.

The unit would certainly need a massive grant to start with. Subsequent income would depend on the use made of the service. If one reckons that 12,000 postgraduates sit examinations each year, and undergraduates sit about 40,000 distinct examinations at M.B. level (quite apart from class examinations) the cost of the service begins to come into perspective. Of course even a nominal charge might seem expensive to the universities, though in terms of staff time saved it is probably good business. But for economical operation one must reckon on nearly all the examining bodies agreeing to join the service. Since overheads would be very much heavier than costs of handling papers, the more bodies who opt out of the service the higher the cost to those who use it. It is clearly an exercise whose financial viability is a matter for the most anxious consideration, but for which the main requirement is use by a very high proportion of the possible field. There exists of course the possibility of export of services to some of the less developed countries, but one cannot count on much profit from that.

What would users expect to get out of it?: either a complete paper according to specifications, or a choice of questions from which the examiners could make a choice of questions; where necessary, advice on the conduct of the examination, and practice material in which the candidates could learn the techniques; after the examination, a return-of-post set of scores and question analyses; according to a standard system but modified by agreement to suit local circumstances. When asked for, such information as the service could give without individual identification of schools as to the relative performance of the candidates in comparison with standards in the rest of the country. And, of course, and perhaps most important, the assurance that the questions had been worked over thoroughly by experts, and that their performance was being thoroughly analysed at all stages.

The process of making questions would of course be a vital one. What we envisage is the formation for each subject of a central panel of perhaps six people who would be the final arbiters. To them would be attached, for perhaps a year at a time, groups of people working in the subject whose job would be to invent new questions and to help the panel to polish them, then to lie fallow for a number of years before serving again. As a corrective to the tendency to over-centralization produced by the central unit, it is absolutely essential that membership of the panels should be evenly distributed through the country.

The questions produced by the panel would be taken over by the central unit and introduced into examinations. Their performance would be most carefully vetted, and considered by the panel and discussed perhaps with both the original contributors and with users. The result ought to be questions of guaranteed soundness and measured difficulty. It is to be assumed that the questions will be held on a computer file. Ultimately, it could even be possible for the entire process to be automatic—given a specification of subject range and standard of difficulty, the entire question paper might be chosen and printed out automatically and the whole process of setting and marking the paper be taken over by the computer. It is unlikely of course that this height of perfection—or absurdity, as one chooses to regard it—will ever be exactly attained. But it is a worth-while goal to attempt to automate as much of the process as we reasonably can. We would repeat again that even if the M.C.Q. part of the examination were entirely automated, this would not involve loss of control by the local examiners. It would be up to them to accept, reject, or modify the paper offered to them in whole or part. It would be up to them to make the decision as to pass or fail. The service would provide them with an efficient measuring instrument: it would be up to them to interpret the measurements in human terms of the worth of the candidates.

A central service would be a failure, however, if it was not a focus for research, both into methods of assessment and into medical education in general. Probably in the early years it would be too busy developing its own techniques to initiate much new work of its own. But it ought to be able at a very early stage to collaborate with others in need of technical advice and assistance in the running of experiments in medical education and assessment. Properly used, it should help to ensure that the computer becomes as successful a tool of medical educational research as it has in so many other research fields.

REFERENCES

ANDERSON, J. (1970), in *Lennox, B., and Lever, Rosemary S.* (1970).

FLINN, R. M. (1970), in *Lennox, B., and Lever, Rosemary S.* (1970).

GIBBONS, J. L., and WOOD, W. ANNE (1970), in *Lennox, B., and Lever, Rosemary S.* (1970).

HARRIS, F. T. C., and BUCKLEY-SHARP, M. D. (1968), 'Automation of Multiple-choice Examination Marking', *Br. J. med. Educ.*, **2**, 48.

— — — — (1970), in *Lennox, B., and Lever, Rosemary S.* (1970).

HUBBARD, J. P., and CLEMENS, W. V. (1961), *Multiple Choice Examinations in Medicine*. Philadelphia: Lea & Febiger.

IVES, J. (1970), in *Lennox, B., and Lever, Rosemary S.* (1970).

LENNOX, B., and DUFF, CHRISTINE (1966), 'A Trial of Computer Marking of Medical Students' Examinations using Lector', in *Computers in the Hospital Service* (ed. BROWN, W. A.), p. 70. Glasgow: Western Regional Hospital Board.

— — and LEVER, ROSEMARY S. (1970), 'Seminar on Machine Marking of Medical Multiple Choice Question Papers', *Br. J. med. Educ.*, **4,** 219.

— — and WALLACE, AGNES A. C. (1970), 'Use of Computers in Assessment of Medical Students', *Scott. med. J.*, **15,** 400.

LEVER, ROSEMARY S., HARDEN, R. M., WILSON, G. M., and JOLLEY, J. L. (1970), 'A Simple Answer Sheet Designed for Use with Objective Examinations', *Br. J. med. Educ.*, **4,** 37.

OWEN, S. G., ROBSON, MARGARET G., SANDERSON, P. H., SMART, G. A., and STOKES, J. F. (1967), 'Experience of Multiple Choice Question Examination for Part 1 of the M.R.C.P.', *Lancet*, **2,** 1034.

DISCUSSION

Question (Professor W. I. Card): What kind of correlation coefficient does one find between two sets of M.C.Q. papers set to the same 100 students ?

Answer: Up to about 0.85 and not often under 0.75. This is a good deal better than with essays, vivas or practical examinations. However, if you set several essays, their performance improves.

Question (Professor W. I. Card): Does one find in your results a normal distribution of scores ?

Answer: Usually approximately normal. In fact, often normal when one would not expect it to be, as in groups of students from whom an earlier examination might be expected to have removed the bottom tail.

Question (Dr. H. Summers): I am unhappy about the type of multiple choice of questions asked. One has to realize that students may wish to qualify their answers apart from answering 'yes' or 'no'.

Answer: No questions are asked requiring qualification. Students with most knowledge obtain most marks. This idea of allowing students to indicate their degree of certainty is an attractive one, but it is really more use as a method of research into student attitudes than as an everyday examination procedure. There will always be a fringe of questions between the ones he knows with reasonable certainty and the ones of which he is completely ignorant, but with a well set paper and a proper marking system, what distinguishes the good students from the poor students is the number of questions to which they can give a confident answer.

Question (Dr. H. Summers): Since most medical students are on the whole inarticulate in writing, the absence of essay questions would surely be a step in the wrong direction.

Answer: Though the multiple choice question (M.C.Q.) is the best single type of examination, other tests are also available requiring knowledge on the part of students how to write essays or read the literature.

An examination has two functions: one, the immediate one, to put candidates in order; the other, propagandist and educational, to demonstrate to the student what you think it is important to know. M.C.Q. is the best single method for the first. Various other methods can be used for the second. Essays help to convince the students that they need to remain literate. But a better way is to give each student a subject and give him a term or more in which to find out about it and write it up properly. He will learn a great deal from that. You will find it very hard to mark the results, but there is no doubt of the educational value of the process.

Question (Professor F. W. Donaldson): When do you eliminate a bad question ?

Answer: Roughly speaking, when less than 10 per cent of the students get it right or more than 90 per cent. Also if the discrimination index is very poor and there is no obvious reason for this, though I don't think this is as good a reason if the question seems otherwise a good one. Also if the facts alter or it becomes irrelevant to our teaching programme.

Question (Dr. H. Summers): What would happen if there had been some very recent new discoveries in a subject which candidates knew about and the examiner did not ?

Answer: Of course, this can happen. It has happened to me. But it is again not likely to involve more than one question in a whole paper, and will not affect the results. There is also a built-in machinery for uncovering it. If the top students all get a question wrong and the bottom students all get it right, something odd is happening which needs investigation and the event suggested is one of the possible causes. And, of course, the whole process is open to inspection. One's fellow examiners will have seen the paper beforehand, and they ought between them to spot any such error on the part of the compiler. Everything the examiner does is open to inspection and criticism by other examiners. With an essay question, the question itself may be a good one but the examiner's premises for marking it may be completely false, and there is no easy way of finding out if this is so.

Question (Dr. H. Summers): What should a candidate do when faced with an ambiguous question, such as that shown on the screen during the lecture?

Answer: The question shown on the screen is admittedly a poor one. It was constructed simply by modifying the stem of a one-from-five and the result is a poor 'grouped true-false'. My text does, in fact, note its imperfection, though I omitted this in delivery. One would modify the question if it was to be used in practice—one must try and produce questions for which there is no such ambiguity. However, a few such bad questions will not ruin the whole examination. What matters in scoring is not the individual questions, but the total, and a student who is good enough to spot the flaws in such questions will be able in compensation to answer all the easier questions that his weaker colleagues find difficult.

Question (Dr. O. Fokkens): Is it not true that even after you have done all the computer analyses, and the figures have indicated a good question, it may still be a very poor question?

Answer: Of course this is true. You must ask questions about the right kind of thing. A question that tests intelligence or general knowledge will usually be done better by the top half of the class than by the bottom half, and may have excellent indices and yet be entirely irrelevant to the subject of the examination. There is no substitute for common sense in these things.

PANEL DISCUSSION*
(J. M. Rawles; J. Emlyn Jones; A. Fleck; H. Summers; B. D. Young; B. Lennox)

Question (Dr. R. Ward): With foresight, what equipment would you recommend when setting up a 4-bedded intensive care unit?

Answer (Dr. J. Rawles): Buy the cheapest and simplest oscilloscope and spend the rest on nurses' salaries and more staff.

Question (Dr. A. Fernandez): Do you plan to put the system on-line?

Answer (J. Emlyn Jones): Yes, particularly the cytology and blood transfusion work. But I am not sure what time we shall cover (8 hours; 6 hours; emergencies?).

Question (Professor F. W. Donaldson): What is the cost per patient per day of on-line arrangements? In the U.S.A. it is between $7 and $10,

---

* At the end of the second day's proceedings.

10 per cent of the total cost and 25 per cent of the running cost of a hospital and clerical help).

Answer (J. Emlyn Jones): I don't know. I don't think there is an on-line computer system in a U.K. hospital at present.

Question (Professor B. Lennox): Surely whatever may be the difficulties of deciding whether the major schemes, and particularly the on-line schemes, can be justified in purely financial terms, there is a great deal of work in the way of large scale transfer of relatively simple items of information that occurs in hospitals where there is very little doubt that computerization would be justifiable. I mean, particularly, the relatively simple administrative and statistical data.

Answer (J. Emlyn Jones): I have no reliable information. Even with a sound computer system most of the present expenditure will continue; there may be even additional expenditure.

Question (Professor F. W. Donaldson): By 1980 hospital expenses in the U.S.A. will have increased considerably (probably from $100 million to $10,000 million), while the cost of hardware will be reduced. However, there is no other way but computerization.

Answer (J. Emlyn Jones): In 1950 expenditure in Manchester was about £14 million; it is now £85 million, and by 1980 may well be £150 million. But I don't think this is the problem. Hardware costs are certainly coming down, but computer support costs (programmers, etc.) are increasing. We spent £200,000 on hardware, while support now costs £120,000. I don't know what the cost of support will be in 1980.

Question (E. C. Sirey): It is suggested that the cost of software should be spread over several systems in order to reduce the expense for a given system.

Answer (J. Emlyn Jones): I am somewhat cynical about the spread of software costs; I think that total expenditure on software tends to remain high because software and software packages don't remain constant but are continually subject to amendment and improvement.

Comment (Dr. A. Fleck): Everybody wants to modify software for their own system, because standard software does not apply.

Question (E. C. Sirey): Is it desirable to get the same software for different hospitals ?

Answer (Dr. A. Fleck): Almost every laboratory with the Elliott 903 system has its own programmer. Local modifications seem to be essential.

Question (Dr. A. Fernandez): I would like to know the cost of the following: Computer, hardware device, interfacing of the PDP computers and IBM 1130 software. I would also wish to know the identity of those who have linked an AutoAnalyser with a computer.

Answer (Dr. A. Fleck): In general, I believe Aberdeen has spent about £30,000 on a digital PDF12 system, while Glasgow has rented an IBM 1130 system. The total capital cost works out at approximately £40,000. The Elliott B system costs about £35,000, and the A system about £50,000. The cost of interfacing hardware depends on how it is done. Costs of interfacing are difficult to assess since the cost of the ADC may be included in the cost of the computer. The cost of the Min Mac chart reader is approximately £2500.

Question (*Dr. O. Fokkens*): What is the opinion of the panel about producing a wholly integrated information system in a hospital?

Answers (*Dr. H. Summers*): No comment.

(*J. Emlyn Jones*): Negative answer for the near future, partly positive in the long run (about 25 years say).

(*Dr. J. Rawles*): No comment.

(*B. D. Young*): It is better to go for a small machine. It is difficult to judge, particularly since during the two days of the Symposium we were dealing with different machines.

(*Professor B. Lennox*): Our own philosophy at the Glasgow Western Infirmary (and I think it is generally true of Scotland as a whole and of the policy of its Advisory Committee) is to exploit local strengths: to take individual schemes where there is a demonstrable need, and keenness and expertise among the people on the spot, and to develop them to the point where they are capable of standing on their own feet; and to regard linkage of them together into a unified system as a second stage. We have, however, in our own scheme at the Western Infirmary a provision that should make ultimate unification considerably easier. We intend to establish what we call a Patient Register, basically a file of minimal data on all in-patients, which will serve to mechanize some of the functions of the records office, and look after waiting lists and follow-ups, and to provide administrative data such as a local and up-to-date H.A.A. We intend it to serve also as a central exchange for all information about patients, to which separate departments will be connected as they become computerized one by one. In this way the one major constraint on the independence of design of each separate scheme will be the need to be able to communicate with the Register. This seems to us to be a reasonable approach to a compromise between total computerization in one shot and complete fragmentation.

Closing address

J. Rose

In the absence of the President, The Lord Rosenheim, who had to leave today to attend an important debate on smoking in the House of Lords, it fell upon me to close this Symposium; no doubt, his Lordship would have done this much better than I. Lord Rosenheim asked me to convey his apologies to all present and his regrets at not being able to address you at the end of the Symposium.

During the last two days we have been treated to a critical and comprehensive review of the use of computers in medicine in a wide sense. While the first Symposium held in 1968 was concerned with methodology and the problems of areas where computers could be used, the present event dealt with the practical uses, and the general theme was how to use these machines for better medical services and more effective utilization of resources. Above all, the emphasis was on a critical appraisal of the art. This was evident in the discussions following the lectures and each day's work. While opinions appeared to be somewhat polarized, the theme of practical and possible applications was very much in evidence.

The success of this event was due in no small measure to the efforts of all involved in the preliminary work. I wish to pay particular tribute to the deputy organizer, Dr. J. H. Mitchell, for his unstinting support and many valuable suggestions; without his assistance this Symposium would have hardly achieved the high standard and usefulness. My thanks are also due to Dr. H. Summers for his splendid assistance, and the secretary, Miss R. R. Black, for her important contribution to the organization and running of the event. You have all seen her in action, and the smoothness of the proceedings was due to a large extent to her skill and hard work put in both before and during the Symposium. May I also thank Professor Donaldson for his kind offer to travel from the U.S.A. in order to deliver his lecture and participate in the proceedings, particularly in view of the considerable financial sacrifices involved. A great debt of gratitude is due to the Chairmen of the Sessions and the Lecturers for their splendid cooperation. I must not forget to thank the audience for their profound attention and eagerness to participate in the discussions. Finally, may I, on your behalf, thank Lord Rosenheim for his kindness in presiding at the Symposium and official dinner; he has, indeed, invested this Symposium with dignity and eminence.

We have now reached the end of the two-day event. It is hoped that you have all enjoyed the proceedings and company. Perhaps we shall meet again in three years' time, as suggested by our President, but without the difficulties engendered by the prolonged postal strike or other disruptive factors which have depleted our numbers and increased the preparatory work. Let us hope that the projected third Symposium will be an even greater success than the present one.